Mediterranean Diet and Health:
Current News and Prospects

ISBN 2-7420-0343-6

Éditions John Libbey Eurotext
127, avenue de la République, 92120 Montrouge, France
Tel: 01.46.73.06.60
Fax: 01.40.84.09.99
e-mail: contact@john-libbey-eurotext.fr
Website: http://www.john-libbey-eurotext.fr

John Libbey and Company Ltd
163-169 Brompton Road, Knightsbridge
London SW3 IPY, England
Tel.: (44) (0) 23 80 65 02 08

John Libbey CIC
Corso Trieste 42
00198 Roma, Italia
Tel.: (39) 06 841 2673

© 2001, John Libbey Eurotext, Paris.

This work may not be reproduced, partially or in its entirety, without the authorisation of the editor or of the Centre Français d'Exploitation du Droit de Copie, 20 rue des Grands-Augustins, 75010 Paris.

Mediterranean Diet and Health: Current News and Prospects

Pierre Besançon

Stéphane Debosque

Francis Delpeuch

Bernard Descomps

Mariette Gerber

Claude-Louis Léger

Martine Padilla

Marc Puygrenier

Foreword: Anna Ferro-Luzzi

Work co-ordinated by AGROPOLIS-Montpellier-France

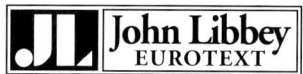

Mediterranean Diet and Health

Table of contents

List of authors	VII
Presentation of the work *Jacques Blanc, Former Minister, President of the Languedoc-Roussillon Region*	IX
Introduction *Daniel Constantin, Prefect of the Languedoc-Roussillon Region*	XI
Foreword *Anna Ferro-Luzi, from the National Nutrition Institute – Roma (Italy)*	XIII
I – Epidemiology	
1. Health benefits of the Mediterranean consumption model *Mariette Gerber- INSERM-CRLC*	3
II – Nutritional contribution of food in the Mediterranean consumption model	
2. Olive oil, olive oil by-products and olive fruit: current data and developments concerning the food and health relationship *Claude-Louis Léger, Bernard Descomps – Université Montpellier I – Medicine*	53
3. Fish and sea foods *Mariette Gerber, Luçay Han-Ching, Gérard Pieroni – INSERM, CRLC, IFREMER*	69
4. Wine consumption and cardiovascular disease prevention *Claude-Louis Léger, Marie-Annette Carbonneau, Bernard Descomps – Université Montpellier I – Medicine*	77
5. Beneficial effects of fruits and vegetables on health *Pierre Besançon – Université Montpellier II – Science and Technologies*	93
Technical information	
Polyphenols: an introduction *Claude-Louis Léger, Marie-Josephe Amiot-Carlin – INRA Avignon*	103
Food fibre: nutritional interest in human diet *Denis Lairon – Inserm U476-Marseille*	109

III – Eating behaviour and culinary practices

6. Eating behaviour and culinary practices
Martine Padilla, Françoise Aubaille-Sallenave, Bénédicte Oberti – CIHEAM-IAM M, French National Natural History Museum 113

IV – Prospects for Mediterranean food

7. Preserve the health capital of food with appropriate technological treatments
Pierre Besançon – Université Montpellier II – Science and Technologies 131

8. New agricultural practices and agro-food innovation to develop the health value of Mediterranean food
Stéphane Debosque, Marc Puygrenier – Regional Agricultural Chamber of Languedoc-Rousillon, Agropolis 139

9. Preserving and promoting the Mediterranean diet for health: towards integrated nutrition policies
Francis Delpeuch – IRD 149

Glossary of scientific and technical terminology 161

Index 165

List of authors

Anna Ferro-Luzzi: Professor – Director of the National Nutrition Institute – Rome – Italy Wrote the foreword of this collective work.

Authors:

Pierre Besançon: Professor-Université Montpellier 11-ISIM – Laboratoire de Génie Biologique et Sciences de l'Aliment. Unité de Nutrition – 34095 Montpellier cedex 05.

Stéphane Debosque: Director of the Regional Agriculture Chamber Languedoc – Roussillon-Maison des Agriculteurs-Mas de Saporta – 34970 Lattes.

Francis Delpeuch: Director of the Laboratoire de Nutrition Tropical-Département Sociétés et Santé-UR7-IRD-91 1, avenue Agropolis – BP 5045 – 34032 Montpellier Cedex 1.

Bernard Descomps: Professor – Université Montpellier I-Directeur du Laboratoire de Nutrition Humaine et Athérogenèse – Institut de Biologie – boulevard Henry IV – 34060 Montpellier.

Mariette Gerber: MD, PhD, Sc D, Head of Metabolic Epidemiology Group, Cancer Research Cancer, – CRLC-INSERM, 34298 Montpellier Cedex 5.

Claude-Louis Léger: Research Director – Université Montpellier 1 – Laboratoire de Nutrition Humaine et Athérogenèse – Institut de Biologie – boulevard Henry IV – 34060 Montpellier.

Martine Padilla: Doctor – Scientific Administrator of the CIHEAM – IAM.M-Département de Recherche Marchés et Sécurité Alimentaire – Institut Agronomique Méditerranéen-3191, route de Mende – 34093 Montpellier Cedex 5.

Marc Puygrenier: Doctor – Director of Valorisation – Agropolis, avenue Agropolis, 34394 Montpellier Cedex 5.

Also contributed:

Marie-Josephe Amiot-Carlin: Doctor-Research Director – INRA – Station de Technologie des Produits Végétaux – Domaine Saint-Paul –Site Agroparc – 84914 Avignon Cedex 9.

Françoise Aubaile Sallenave: Doctor-Chargée de Recherche CNRS – Laboratoire d'Ethnobiologie: "Appropriation et socialisation de la nature". URA 882 CNRS – Museum National d'Histoire Naturelle – 43, rue Cuvier – 75231 Paris Cedex 5.

Marie-Annette Carbonneau: Doctor – Université Montpellier 1 – Laboratoire de Nutrition Humaine et Athérogenèse – Institut de Biologie – boulevard Henry IV – 34060 Montpellier.

Luçay Han-Ching: Doctor – Head of "product valorisation" department IFREMER-Centre de Nantes – rue de l'Ile-d'Yeu – BP 21 105 – 44311 Nantes Cedex 3.

Denis Lairon: Research Director – Director of the INSERM Unit U 476 – Centre Viton – 18 avenue Mozart – 13009 Marseille.

Bénédicte Oberti: Doctor, IAMM, Département de Recherche Marchés et Sécurité Alimentaire – Institut Agronomique Méditerranéen-3191, route de Mende – 34093 Montpellier Cedex 5.

Gérard Piéroni: Doctor – Unité Nutrition Humaine et lipides: Biodisponibilité, métabolisme et régulation – INSERM U 476 – Centre Viton – 18 avenue Mozart – 13009 Marseille.

Presentation of the work

As a doctor and the President of a region where agriculture, Mediterranean products, wine growing and agro-food play a major role in the economy and regional development, I became personally involved in the recognition of the beneficial effects of the Mediterranean diet.

The scientific community of the Languedoc-Roussillon is also highly mobilised, *via* two major excellence scientific research centres: biology-health and agronomy.

In this collective work, answers are provided to questions everyone asks oneself: what are the effects of Mediterranean diet on health? What do medicine and agronomy experts think about this? What is the current status of knowledge in this field? What research merits to be continued or started in order to better know and better understand the interest of "better eating", for its immediate pleasure, well-being and the long-lasting preservation of health?

All these questions are currently part of a true public debate.

I thank each and everyone for their participation in the collective thinking and wish that this scientific initiative will contribute to develop the attraction of our Mediterranean products.

Jacques Blanc
Former Minister
President of the Languedoc-Roussillon Region

Introduction

From a scientific point of view there is an objective relationship between diet and health.

Throughout time, life habits and specially eating habits have been regulated successively by religious authorities (fasting, food forbidden by dietary law, etc.), then by the medical profession, while the structuring of food science only takes place at the beginning of the xxth century with the appearance of dietetics which aims at restoring the major metabolic balance, then closer to our time, the advent of nutrition as a research field of its own and finally in the last few years the promotion of food to a medicine status, "food-drug".

Mediterranean diet, beyond the epidemiological surveys and the French paradox, appears as one of the best adapted to the maintenance of good health, reconciling nutritional interest and organoleptic quality, combined with life habits which go further than just the control of diet.

Traditionally, Mediterraneans had a considerable and varied consumption of food of vegetable origin, ate little red meat, fish, very little milk and butter, but fresh cheese and yoghurt instead; they added lipids almost exclusively in the form of olive oil, and finally consumed red wine, moderately with meals... (as recommended by common sense!)

However, can this eating habit be exported to other regions and other cultures?

This questions merits in-depth study, and is the objective of this work.

Researchers decided to take stock of the knowledge on Mediterranean diet in order to valorise the achievements.

Agro-food companies will be able to obtain new commercial arguments. As for consumers, they will have better information in order to make choices in the context of healthy and balanced life habits.

It is a strategic work for our region and for its economical development.

Daniel Constantin
Prefect of the Languedoc-Roussillon Region

Foreword

THE MEDITERRANEAN DIET: DO WE KNOW ALL WE NEED TO KNOW?

The Mediterranean Diet is part and parcel of a way of life, handed down to us from our grandparents, that has enjoyed over the years a growing popularity world-wide. The most endearing features of this style of life have been a combination of a temperate climate, the beauty of the land and the fragrance of its products, a close-knitted enlarged family structure, a relaxed tempo of everyday life, the social significance of the meals and – of course – the celebrated Mediterranean Diet. The latter has acquired a well deserved recognition not only with the "gourmets", but also with the scientific community thanks to its health-protective potential. This highly promising connotation of the Mediterranean Diet was first revealed by Professor Ancel Keys, an eminent scientist and an epidemiologist of world renown who, on the basis of his findings from the Seven Country Study, wrote in 1975 the book "How to eat well and stay well the Mediterranean way" which remained on the best seller list till now. Since then, many epidemiological, clinical, metabolic and experimental studies have been conducted in the effort to precisely pinpoint the composition of the Mediterranean Diet and to identify the mechanisms by which it reduces the risk for cardiovascular disease as well as – as it became evident later on – for cancer. The earlier emphasis, exclusively placed on its fat moiety and the lipid hypothesis of the cardiovascular disease, was later expanded to include the oxidative hypothesis. This triggered off extensive investigations on the antioxidant nutrients present in the diet, and it was soon established that indeed the Vitamin E and Vitamin C of the diet contributed significantly to lowering the dietary risk factor for cardiovascular disease. On the other hand, it soon became clear that a consistent proportion of the variance of the risk still remained to be explained.

While studies were being conducted to provide scientific evidence on the importance of the various ingredients of the diet, it became apparent that remarkably little was known, besides and beyond its lipid composition, about which foods did actually compose the Mediterranean Diet. This gap in the knowledge is regretful as it has represented a major obstacle for a rapid progress in the understanding of the health-promoting attributes afforded by that particular dietary style. The Mediterranean Diet was in no way condified and, even now, it is difficult to decide which is, or was, its composition. So for example, while everyone agrees that olive oil is the main if not unique source of dietary fats, it appears that while the Cretans consumed in the early '60s no less than 100 g/day olive oil, the Italians fared as well with just about half that amount. In terms of percent energy, these amount respectively to 42% energy from total fat in Crete and less than 30% in Italy. Considering the risk that the energy density of the diet may represent in relation to obesity, one wonders the wisdom of currently advising the population that they need not limit the amount of olive oil in their diet, as long as it is olive oil. Should we not adjust the advice to the changing and increasingly sedentary modern life style, and drop the percent of fat energy from the Greek to the Italian level? Interestingly, other dietary surveys conducted in the '30s and 40's in Italy reveal that an even lower amount of dietary fat was consumed in those years, and that such low consumption of fat was not linked to poverty, as also richer socio-economic urban classes consumed similar amounts of fat. This seems to suggest that the modern tendency of the "western" consumer to favour high fat foods might derive more from technological circumstances created by the food industry than from an innate tendency of the consumer.

The pristine Medirerranean Diet was characterised also by the high proportion of plant food, with ample reliance on low extraction rate cereal flours – the major dietary staple, which contributed in the early 30's up to 65% of the total energy of the diet of Sicilian peasants; large amounts of vegetables were also present. Both are rich source of polyphenols. This vast and varied family of polyphenolic compounds is no more considered to be an inert component of the diet, that escapes digestion in the human intestine and that is important only because it imparts colour, flavour, astringency and so on, to our foods. There is ample consensus that these compounds might variously contribute to the beneficial effects of the Mediterranean Diet, acting as antioxidants, phytoestrogens, chelators of metals, activators or inhibitors of enzymes and so on. But there are still many gaps in the proper understanding of these aspects, possible synergysms or antagonisms, bioavailability, and even the amounts that are present in the foods. The type and amounts of these compounds present in any given fruit is greatly influenced by a wide number of factors, such as agricultural practices, exposure of the plant to infections and parasites, the degree of ripeness, the nature of technological process undergone by the fruit, whether it is pealed or not, and many other more. There are also emerging issues with unknown compositional and/or functional implications for foods which have traditionnaly belonged to the Mediterranean culture. It is yet too early to appreciate what might be the consequence of the substitution of traditionally grown Southern European fruit and vegetables with their genetically modified counterparts. There are possible pleiotropic effects induced by a particular modification and subtle unintentional changes may take place in the composition of a vegetable. The current approach to establishing the substantial equivalence of GMO products does not take into account, or only to a very limited extent, the large variety of polyphenols that are normally present in the Mediterranean Diet.

It appears therefore that there is much ground still to cover before a coherent picture of the health impact of the Mediterranean diet and its mechanism are fully understood. A book like the present one, collecting under one title an update of the scientific progress in a variety of disciplines ranging from agricultural practices to food technology, from epidemiology to policy, is an important step in that direction.

Anna-Ferro Luzzi
National Institute of Nutrition
Rome, Italy

Epidemiology

Health benefits of the Mediterranean consumption model

Mariette Gerber

It has been more than ten years since epidemiological studies, especially the Seven Countries Study (Keys, 1986) mentioned the health benefit related to Mediterranean diet. However, it took the publication of studies carried out in English-speaking and Scandinavian countries, epidemiology's preferred stamping ground, in order for the health benefit concept of Mediterranean diet to come back.

Therefore, this hypothesis was strengthened by its contrary, not only in a geographical sense, from the North to the South, but also on a conceptual level. Indeed, the relation to diseases was studied on a food by food and even nutrient by nutrient basis, while it seems more and more likely that an overall vision of Mediterranean habits is required to grasp all the advantages.

This analytical approach corresponds to the usual scientific method, which allows the demonstration of the cause effect relationships and mechanisms. Therefore, we will see initially the limits of this approach in an epidemiology context, briefly mentioning the epidemiological methods and difficulties encountered to prove a cause effect relationship.

Then the relationship to pathologies will be carried out on a food basis, introducing the nutrients found in the food to suggest the mechanisms. We will see how the sources of these nutrients are intricate, especially with respect to plant origin food *(figure 1)*.

In the conclusion we will try to identify the reasons in favour of a holistic concept of the Mediterranean diet.

EPIDEMIOLOGY. THEORETICAL SUMMARY

Epidemiology is the study of pathological disorders at the level of one or several populations. It is divided into **descriptive epidemiology**, which indicates how a disease is distributed in a set of populations *(figure 2)*, and **analytical epidemiology** that tries to identify the risk factors of these diseases. Two types of studies allow such research: **case-control studies** compare the exposure to risk factors of subjects with a characterised disease and that of controls; the latter are ideally similar on all points except for the presence of the disease. These studies

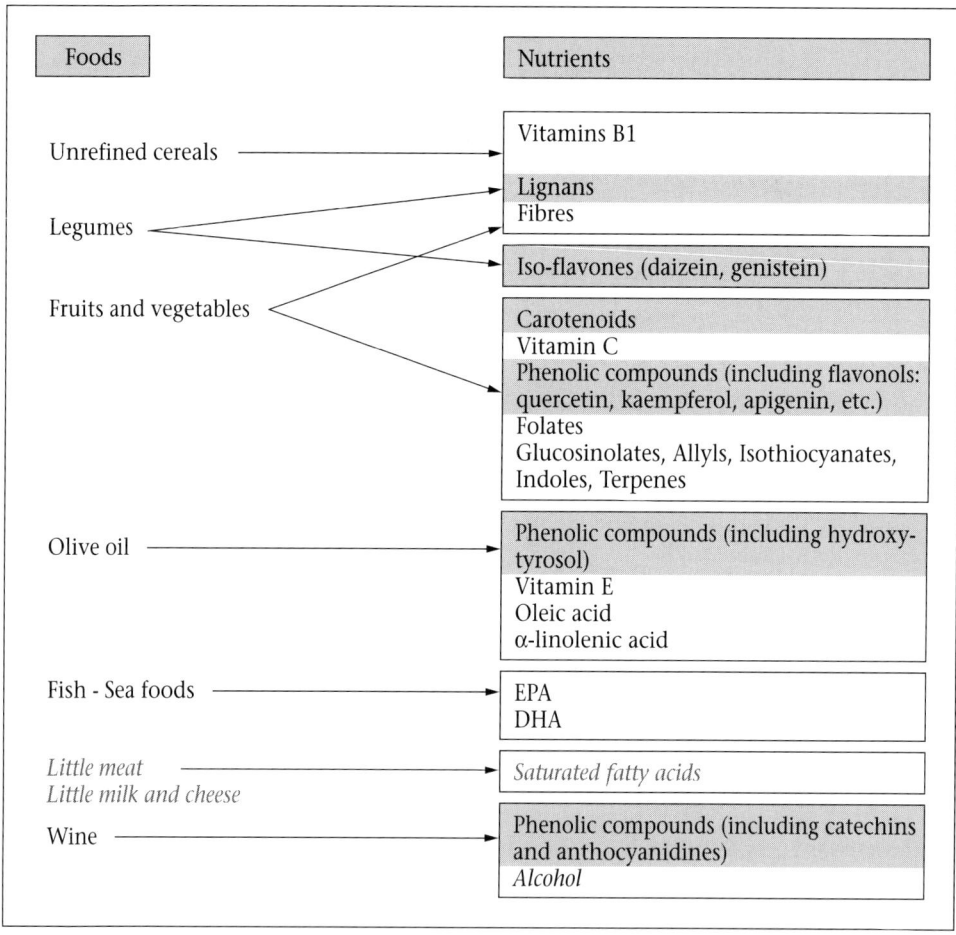

Figure 1. Source of nutrients with respect to plant origin food.

are generally retrospective, *i.e.* the subjects must remember their previous exposure to the risk factors. It can be easily conceived that this method would be affected by errors especially when the food consumption of the past must be evaluated. For this reason **prospective studies** are generally preferred. In these studies a population set (example: a cohort of nurses, a cohort of gas or electricity company employees, etc.) is questioned in the beginning of the study about its usual food consumption and other risk factors (smoking, physical activity, other exposures, etc.). These surveys are carried out using a questionnaire, most often a consumption frequency questionnaire, to evaluate the usual food intake. Biological food markers can also be measured in various body tissues. The cohort is followed over a certain number of years to record the incidence of diseases. Finally, intervention studies can be employed which are supposed to provide the proof of a cause effect relationship between a nutritional intake and a disease, by comparing the incidence or mortality in two population

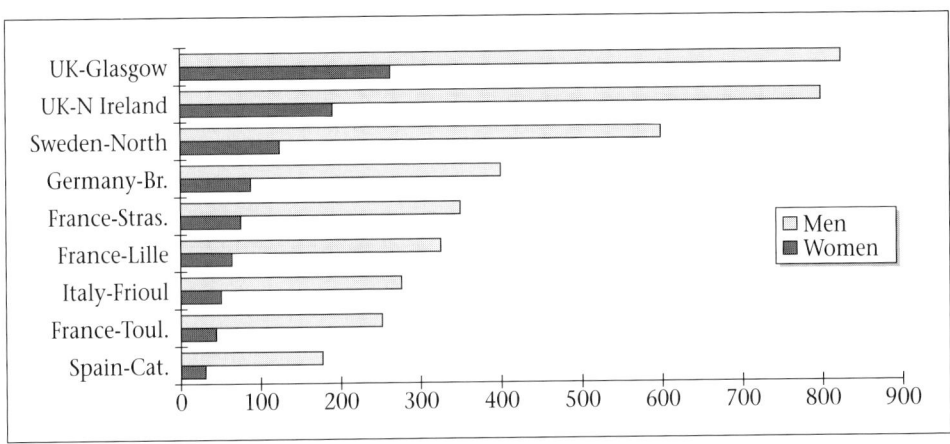

Figure 2A. Incidence of coronary heart disease per 100,000.

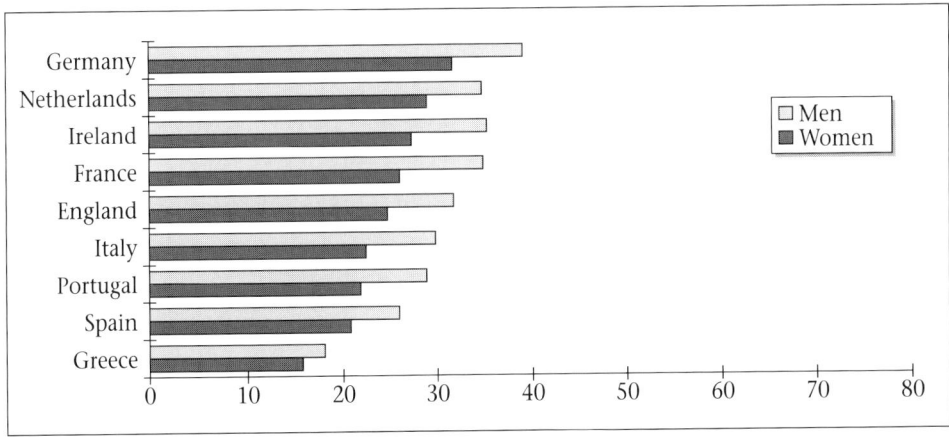

Figure 2B. Colo-rectal cancer: incidence standardised for age per 100,000.

stamples, one treated with the nutrient studied and the other with a placebo. The major intervention studies published in the last few years and mentioned in the text are presented in *Table I*.

The relationship between exposure to a certain factor (for example the consumption of fat) and the occurrence of the disease is calculated in the same way for the three types of studies. The probability of the appearance of the disease as a function of the level of exposure to the factor considered is obtained. This is expressed by the *Odds Ratio* (OR).

Table I. Major intervention studies

Authors/countries	Subjects	Treatment	Follow-up	Criteria
LINXIAN 1 China Biot et al., 1993	29,584 general population in Linxian completion: 93%	C: vit C+ molybdenum 120 mg + 30 µg D: β-carotene + vit E, + Se 15 mg + 30 mg + 50 mg plasma level 1,5 µmol/L (14.5x)	5 years and 3 months	All causes of mortality, all cancers
LINXIAN 2 China Li et al., 1993	3,318 subjects with oesophageous dysplasia from the preceding cohort	14 vitamins + 12 minerals at 2-3 x RDA among which β-carotene, (15 mg/jour), vit A, E, 60 IU, C, 180 mg, B1, B2, B6, B12, folic acid, biotin, Ca, Se, Mb, Zn, Mn, I, Cu, Fe	6 years	Oesophageal and gastric cardia cancers mortality and incidence
LINXIAN 3 China Mark et al., 1994	same study as Linxian 2	id	6 years	Regression of oesophageal dysplasia
ATBC Finland The ATBC cancer prevention study group, 1994	29,000 smokers completion: 93% drop-out: 31%	1-β-carotene 20 mg/jour plasma levels: 5.3 µmol/l (17.6x) 2-vit. E 50 mg/day plasma levels: 42.5 µmol/l (1.5x) 3-1+2	5 to 8 years	Incidence of lung cancers and others
CARET United States Omenn et al., 1996	18,314 smokers, ex-smokers, asbestos workers completion: 93% drop-out: 35%	β-carotene 30 mg/day + 25,000 IU vit. A plasma level: 3.6 µmol/l (12.4x)	Average: 4 years	Incidence of lung cancers and others
Physicians' Health Study United States Hennekens et al., 1996	22,071 doctors completion: 78% drop-out: 20%	β-carotene 50 mg/day plasma level: 1.7 µmol/l (4x)	Average: 12 years	Incidence of lung cancer and MCV
Skin Cancer Prevention Study Greenberg et al., 1990; 1996	1,720 subjects with recently removed skin cancer completion: 80%	β-carotene 50 mg/day plasma level: 3,3 µmol/l (10x)	Average 4.3 years	Non-melanoma skin cancers
The Polyp Prevention Study United States Greenberg et al., 1994	864 subjects with sporadic adenomas removed in the 3 previous months completion: 82% drop-out: 13%	1-β-carotene 25 mg/day plasma level: 1.1 µmol/l (2.7x) 2-vitamin C 1 g/day + vit. E 400 mg/day plasma level: 30.6 µmol/l (1.4x) 3-=1+2	4 years	New adenomas
The Australian Polyp Prevention Study Australia Mac Lennan et al., 1995	390 subjects with > 1 polyp removed on day 0 drop-out: 28%	β-carotene 20 mg no information on plasma levels	24 and 48 months	Recurrence of small and large adenomas
CHAOS Great Britain Stephens et al., 1996	2,002 patients MCV diagnosis M+F	400 or 800 IU vit. E plasma level: 51.1 µmol/l	2 years	Non fatal infarction, coronary mortality
GISSI Prev. Invest. Italy 1999	11,234 patients with recent infarction	300 mg vit. E no information on plasma levels	3 and a half years	Non fatal infarction, ictus coronary mortality

> **How to interpret the Odds Ratio (OR)**
>
> To estimate the probability of appearance of a disease, several classes of exposure to the risk factor (in our case a nutrient, a food or a group of foods) are selected and a value is attributed to the reference class of exposure. If the calculation of the OR attributes to a more exposed or less exposed class of subjects a value less than 1, it indicates a lower risk for this class of exposure. If on the contrary a value greater than 1 is obtained, it indicates an increased risk for this exposure class. For example, if in a study on cardiovascular diseases the subjects consuming the least fruit and vegetables are the reference class, the OR will be less than 1 for the subjects who consume lots of fruit and vegetables. If on a study on stomach cancer, the subjects consuming the greatest amount of vitamin C are the reference class, the OR will be greater than 1 for the subjects who consume less. The OR is accompanied by a confidence interval (CI) that does not include the value 1 if the OR is statistically significant. A dose-response effect is also evaluated by the test of trend which, when significant, shows that risk increases with exposure to the risk factor, or inversely decreases with exposure when the factor considered is protective: for example, the more one consumes fruit and vegetable, the lower the risk of developing a cancer.

The diseases we will discuss – chronic degenerative diseases, mainly cardiovascular diseases and cancers – are multifactorial diseases, *i.e.* they are caused or favoured by several factors. For example, in breast cancer all the stages of the reproductive life with an influence on the hormonal system act as a risk factors (late first pregnancy, no or few children, late menopause) to which are associated food factors and direct or susceptibility genetic factors. In order to prove the cause effect relationship between one risk factor and the disease, the possible effect of other factors must be eliminated: for example, the relative risk related to the consumption of fruit and vegetable in cancers is calculated for a constant energy intake. There are statistical methods which allow the control of the effect of confusion factors, *i.e.* factors which vary in the same direction (positively correlated): for example, Mediterraneans combine in their diet many fruits and vegetables and wine as a drink. Therefore, it will be important, in order to estimate the protection related to wine, to use a statistical model that allows the measurement of the effect of wine to a constant consumption of fruit and vegetable: this is adjustment. However, even identifying all the factors, there may remain a residual confusion level, and one is never certain of having identified all the factors, therefore care must be taken in the wording of results. One talks about a an association of observations without being able to affirm that there is cause to effect relationship.

> **Risk factor, risk marker**
>
> A distinction must be made between a risk factor and a risk marker: the first interferes in the causal chain of the disease, for example cholesterol levels in cardiovascular diseases, or colo-rectal adenomas in colon cancer. The second appears as an epi-phenomenon whose causal implication remains to be demonstrated.

As it is difficult to control all the confusion factors, to screen all the errors and correct them, the studies are repeated under different conditions (geography, culture, etc.) with results that may be variable. Criteria defined several years ago (Hill, 1965) are used to evaluate all the studies and reach acceptable conclusions.

Criteria for establishing a causal relationship

– Convergence of results: reproducibility of observations;
– Force of associations: ORs are significant and very different from 1, indicating a high risk probability, for example OR = 2, *i.e.* two times more risk to acquire the disease if exposed to a certain risk factor;
– Dose-effect relationship: existence of a significant test of trend;
– Biological plausibility: is there a biological mechanism likely to explain the effect of the exposure factor. For example, anti-oxidants in fruits and vegetables may oppose the mutagenic action of an oxidative stress in the bronchial or gastric epithelium;
– Analogy/coherence: similarity of observations for diseases with a common physio-pathology (larynx and bronchial cancers).

Based on these criteria a certain number of publications (CNERN, 1996; WRCF, 1997; COMA, 1998; Carotenoids, 1998) or reviews (Ness and Powles, 1996; Kushi *et al.*, 1995; Corpet and Gerber, 1997, Gerber and Corpet, 1997) have been written. This work, combined with the examination of more recent work according to the same criteria, have allowed us to qualify the nature of the link that joins a risk factor and a pathology. Thus one can say that the results are:

– convincing: when they converge to demonstrate either a risk effect, or a protective effect and that a public health measure must follow from this observation;

– probable: when there are some discrepancies, but public health measures must be applied;

– possible: a majority of the studies go in the same direction but the concordance of the results is not sufficient to require a public health measure;

– insufficient: limited, not enough studies to reach a conclusion;

– negative: do not demonstrate a relationship between the disease and the risk factor;

– inconsistent: there are enough studies, but they disagree.

MEDITERRANEAN DIET AND DEGENERATIVE CHRONIC DISEASES

As the Mediterranean diet was traditionally frugal, the entire consumption corresponded to a relatively low energy intake constituted *via* various foodstuffs found in all Mediterranean countries, even though developed in different ways in the different cultures of the Mediterranean countries.

> **Common characteristics of Mediterranean diets**
>
> - High consumption of a variety of fruits and vegetables, fresh and dried, cereals and legumes
> - Use of herbs and spices
> - Low red meat consumption, apart from a little sheep or goat, but fish instead
> - Low consumption of milk and butter, but fresh cheese or yoghurt instead
> - Lipids added almost exclusively as olive oil
> - Red wine consumed in moderation with meals

This type of diet was first associated with a very low risk of cardiovascular diseases and also some types of cancer as shown in *figures 2A and B*, where Mediterranean countries appear grouped at the bottom of the histogram. Other degenerative chronic disorders, such as cataracts, and cognitive ageing could also be modified by such dietary habits.

Each of the characteristics common to the Mediterranean diets led to the study of the relationship between Mediterranean diet and health, *i.e.*:

– plant origin food which covers the fibre intake, anti-oxidants and other interesting micro-components of plants, in a relative low calorie intake;

– animal origin food which allows us to address the – question of fatty acids;

– olive oil;

– red wine in its alcohol and polyphenolic components.

The link between degenerative chronic diseases, essentially cardiovascular diseases and cancers, will be studied within each of the categories.

ENERGETIC FOODS: CALORIC INTAKE

Traditionally it was relatively low (men 2,500 kcal; women 2,000 kcal) in view of the physical activity performed. This is explained by the abundance of low energy density foods (fruit, vegetables, fresh cheese) *versus* high energy density foods (animal products, hard cheeses) which are little consumed. An excess energy intake generally results in excess weight (body mass index, BMI ≥ 25) or obesity (BMI ≥ 30) which are **convincing** risk factors for both cardiovascular diseases and certain cancers: cancer of the kidney, colo-rectal cancer, breast cancer, cancer of the endometrium and to a lesser degree of the ovary and the prostate (the last four cancers are so called hormone-dependent as their growth is favoured by sexual hormones).

How can this similarity of effect for dissimilar diseases be explained? It should be stated that the type of obesity in question corresponds to a particular type: visceral or abdominal obesity, also called android or apple-shaped (*versus* femoro-gluteal obesity, also called gynoid or pear-shaped), and that this type of obesity is characteristic of a metabolic dysfunction syndrome (insulin-resistance syndrome) both on lipids (thus its relationship with cardiovascular diseases), and on sexual hormones (thus its relationship with certain cancers).

> **Insulin-resistance syndrome**
>
> Insulin-resistance and the resulting hyperinsulinemia directly alter fatty acid metabolism, thus the relationship with cardiovascular diseases. Also a decrease in the globulin related to sexual hormones (SHBG) is observed, which induces an increase in testosterone and oestrogen levels, hence the relationship to hormone-dependent cancers. Furthermore, the regulation of another tumour cell growth factor (IGF-1) is altered in this syndrome, which explains that the development of cancers other than hormone-dependent cancers, such as colo-rectal cancer, may be favoured by the insulin-resistance syndrome.

Plant products: lots of fruits, vegetables, herbs, cereals and legumes

Cardiovascular diseases

Foods

Two major reviews (Ness and Powles, 1997 and Law and Morris, 1998) were dedicated to this aspect. Ness and Powles (1997) concluded that all the results demonstrated **convincingly** that fruits and vegetables exerted a strong protective effect against stroke and weaker against coronary diseases. Law and Morris (1998) performed a more critical analysis and quantified the relationship between the fruit and vegetable intake, and the incidence of coronary disease, ischemic accidents and myocardial infarction. Their conclusion is that the risk of ischemic cardiac disease is approximately 15% lower in the 10% of subjects who consume the most fruit and vegetable (*i.e.* more than 600 g/day) than in the 10% who consume the least.

For cereals, the protective effect is probable *(see below under fibres)* when they are not refined (Jacobs *et al.*, 1998; Liu *et al.*, 1999), and for legumes, the results are very limited. There are no specific studies on herbs and spices.

Most of the epidemiological studies consider the nutrients contained in these foods: fibres, vitamins, anti-oxidants, minerals, trying to individualise the effects and mechanisms.

Nutrients

Fibres
They are mostly found in cereals, legumes and to a lesser extent in fruits and vegetables.

Epidemiology
The consumption of fibres is associated with a low risk of cardiovascular diseases in several prospective studies (review in Corpet and Gerber, 1997).

Mechanisms
Fibres have a cholesterol lowering effect: supplementation with oat germ induces a decrease in LDL cholesterol without modifying HDL cholesterol (Swain *et al.*, 1990; Rouanet *et al.*,

> In a Finnish prospective study (Knekt *et al.*, 1994) it was demonstrated that fibres are associated to the low cardiovascular risk in women; this association is not found in men. However, also in Finland, the prospective analysis of the ATBC intervention study described in *Table I* (Pietinene *et al.*, 1996), carried out on 21,930 male smokers, 50 to 60 years old, showed an estimated relative risk (OR) of mortality per coronary disease of 0.69 (0.54 to 0.88) for 34.9 g/day of fibre intake compared to 16.1 g/day. Soluble fibres seemed more effective than insoluble ones. In the Health Professionals Follow-up Study (43,757 men), the fatal and non fatal infarction OR was 0.59 (CI: 0.46 to 0.76) in the fifth consuming the most fibre (28.9 g/day) compared to low consumers (12.9 g/day), the cereal fibres seeming the most "protective" with a decrease of the risk of 29% per 10 g added to the daily intake (Rimm *et al.*, 1996). Finally, two recent studies confirmed the effect of fibres: the Nurses' Health Study in the United States (Wolk *et al.*, 1999) showed that for an increase in consumption of 10 g of fibres, the risk of coronary disease decreases by 19%, the cereal fibres showed the strongest, and that of the Scottish Health Study demonstrated that the effect is seen starting with an intake of 20 g/day (Todd *et al.*, 1999).

1993; Lairon *et al.*, 1996). Also, fibres seem to oppose insulin-resistance (Barnard *et al.*, 1992), which is a risk factor for cardiovascular diseases. Furthermore, recent work (Blache *et al.*, 1999) reported that butyric acid, a short-chain fatty acid whose synthesis is favoured by a large fibre intake, behaves as an anti-oxidant, possibly protecting LDL particle against oxidation.

Anti-oxidants
Except for vitamin E, which is found in almonds, hazelnuts, walnuts and pistachios, and in olive oil (even though at a much lower level than that provided by sunflower oil) the anti-oxidants described below are principally found in fruits and vegetables, herbs and spices and legumes.

Epidemiology
Carotenoids

> **Where are carotenoids found?**
>
> α and β carotenes are found in all red and yellow fruits and vegetables, and also in some cruciferae. More specifically, luteine is found in green leafy vegetables, lycopene in tomatoes and β-cryptoxanthine in oranges.

The results on the protective effect of carotenoids on cardiovascular disease are **inconsistent**.

> Some observation studies have reported a risk reduction in subjects consuming or presenting in their tissues high levels of β-carotene and luteine (Street *et al.*, 1994; Todd *et al.*, 1999) or lycopene and α-carotene (Kohlmeier *et al.*, 1997). However, the clinical results of intervention studies are less convincing: in the 22,000 physicians in the Physician's Health Study *(Table I)* the administration of α-carotene every two days for 12 years did not change the number of cardiovascular accidents, in comparison with the administration of a placebo, and in those who had a pre-existing coronary disease, there was a non-significant increase in cardiovascular mortality (Gaziano *et al.*, 1995). The ATBC intervention study *(Table I)* analysing solely the subjects who had already presented a myocardial infarction showed an increased risk of mortality by coronary accident in the group treated with b-carotene (Rapola *et al.*, 1997).

Vitamin C

There are strong epidemiological indications that allow to say that the reduction of risk of coronary disease by a high intake of vitamin C evaluated by the plasma level is **probable** (Vita *et al.*, 1998; Nyyssonen *et al.*, 1997; Gale *et al.*, 1995; Eichholzer *et al.*, 1992; Todd *et al.*, 1999) even though the effect based on the estimate of the intake by food questionnaire is less conclusive.

> Indeed, it seems that the effect can only be demonstrated if populations with a low intake are studied (Nyyssonen *et al.*, 1997), which would explain the negative studies (Kushi *et al.*, 1996-b; Stampfer *et al.*, 1993; Rimm *et al.*, 1993). Intervention studies examining the effect of vitamin C on coronary heart disease have not been carried out. In the Blot *et al.* (1993) study vitamin C was combined with other nutrients, which does not allow a conclusion on the respective effects of each of the elements *(Table I)*.

Vitamin E

The observation of an inverse relationship between plasma vitamin E levels and coronary disease in 16 European countries (Gey, 1991) was the first to demonstrate the **possible** protective effect of vitamin E. Epidemiological studies based on the ingestion of foods (Knekt, 1994, Kushi *et al.*, 1996) or supplements (Stampfer *et al.*, 1993; Rimm *et al.*, 1993) supported this hypothesis.

> The ABTC intervention study (Rapola *et al.*, 1997, *Table I*) showed that subjects receiving 50 mg/day of α-tocopherol have a lower risk of non-fatal myocardial infarction, but the frequency of these events over the 6 years of follow-up was not significantly different from the placebo group. Only the CHAOS intervention study *(Table I)* showed a beneficial effect of supplementation of vitamin E at high doses (268 mg per day for 510 days) on the incidence of myocardial infarction (but not on mortality) in subjects who had diagnosed signs of cardiovascular disease (Stephens *et al.*, 1996). Vitamin E plasma levels were comparable in the ABTC and CHAOS studies (44.7 vs 51.1 µmol/l). The very recent Italian study (GISSI, 1999) did not show an effect on mortality in subjects supplemented with 300 mg of vitamin E who had presented a myocardial infarction *(Table I)*.

Phenolic compounds

To reconcile the results from the observational epidemiology and intervention studies, it should be reminded that anti-oxidants other than vitamins are present in fruits and vegetables, such as phenolic compounds and in particular flavonoids, and that the b-carotene intake may only be a maker for the consumption of these other constituents. Two prospective studies carried out in the Netherlands (Hertog *et al.*, 1993; Hertog *et al.*, 1995) strongly suggested the importance of these compounds in the reduction of the risk of mortality per cardiovascular disease. These results were confirmed by the prospective study of Knekt *et al.* (1996a) and Yochum *et al.*, (1999), but contradicted by a prospective study carried out in Great Britain (Hertog *et al.*, 1997). Therefore, currently it could be said that the protective effect of these compounds against cardiovascular diseases is **possible**.

Mechanisms

The mechanical transposition of these results was attempted by measuring the level of oxidation of LDL particles and the time of interval of the appearance of oxidised LDL, which are involved in the development of atheroma, in subjects supplemented with β-carotene and vitamins C and E.

In effect, it seems that the protective effect of anti-oxidants does not apply to the early stages of LDL oxidation, but to the already formed atheroma plaque (Diaz *et al.*, 1997). It has been shown that the vitamin E/cholesterol concentration ratio was lower in atheroma plaques than in normal arterial tissues taken on autopsied lesions in 37 subjects, while total vitamin E was higher (Carpenter *et al.*, 1995).

With respect to the phenolic compounds, their availability and their metabolism remain badly known, but it has been demonstrated *ex vivo* that they protect vitamin E contained in LDL particles (Carbonneau *et al.*, 1997 and *technical information* "Polyphenols: an introduction"). Bingham *et al.* (1998) mention in their review that soy-bean containing flavonoids decreases LDL levels, that genistein decreases the activity of tyrosine kinases involved in cellular proliferation, and suppresses the release of NO by inhibition of NO synthetase.

Folic acid

Folic acid (or vitamin B9) is found as folates in many fruits and vegetables (as well as in yeast and liver), and also in legumes plants. Folic acid plasma levels, related to food intake, is inversely correlated to homocysteine plasma levels. Folic acid is required for the transformation of homocysteine into methionine and its deficiency blocks the metabolic route resulting in an accumulation of homocysteine in plasma. In elderly persons high homocysteine concentrations have been observed that could be related to a risk of coronary disease. In the Health's Professionals Follow-up Study (Rimm *et al.*, 1993) men with the highest homocysteine levels in blood had a three-fold greater risk of a myocardial infarction than the other subjects. Apart from the folic acid intake deficiency, it can also be a vitamins B12 and B6 deficiency, since these vitamins are also involved in the accumulation of homocysteine, which explains the results obtained by Rimm *et al.*, (1998) showing a reduction in the risk of coronary disease provided by the concomitant supplementation or dietary intake of folates and vitamin B6 (comparing intakes of 696 μ g and 4.6 μ g/days *vs* 158 μ g and 1.1 μ g/day respectively) than for each on its own. A double blind intervention study carried out with 119 healthy volunteers who consumed cereals with 200 μg of folic acid added or not, for

6 months measured a homocysteine level of 10% less in supplemented subjects (Schorah *et al.*, 1998).

Potassium

Fruits and vegetables are a major source of potassium. Relatively old studies reviewed by Corpet and Gerber (1997) showed that vegetarians have lower blood pressure levels than omnivores; this observation has been confirmed by clinical trials using a potassium supplementation. Therefore, potassium is a probable candidate for cardiovascular risk reduction.

Cancers

Foods

Practically all the epidemiological studies which examined the consumption of fruit and vegetables showed that it was associated with a decrease in cancer risk: 132 studies out of 170 showed a significant protection, *versus* only 6 which showed an increase in the risk. More specifically, based on the publications cited above (CNERNA, 1996; WCRF, 1997; COMA, 1998; IARC, 1998) and more recent studies *(Tables II and III)*, it can be said that the results are **convincing** for all the following types of cancer: upper respiratory-digestive tract, stomach, lung and bronchi; pancreas, cervix and bladder. The effect is only **possible**, and only with respect to vegetables, for hormone-dependent, colon-rectum, kidney and thyroid cancers. The results are **insufficient** or **inconsistent** for the other cancers.

> Some studies have attempted to determine if some vegetables in particular reduced the risk of cancer: the results are **convincing** in the case of tomatoes for oesophageal, stomach and lung cancers, **possible** for oropharyngeal cancers. For most of the other cancers they are **insufficient**. The studies by Giovanucci *et al.* (1995) and Tzonou *et al.* (1999) demonstrating that tomatoes cooked or transformed decreased the risk of prostate cancer should be noted. These studies must be confirmed. In a North American study (Longnecker *et al.*, 1997), carrots and spinach showed an inverse association with breast cancer. Franceschi *et al.*, (1998a) reanalysed all the Italian data. Overall, vegetables seem more protective than fruit among which only the peach/apricot/plum group significantly reduces the risk of cancer of the rectum; apples and fruits rich in vitamin C do not reach significance. All cooked vegetables protect against colon cancer, while only cooked carrots among cooked vegetables significantly reduce the risk of breast cancer. Lettuces and raw carrots reduce the risk of colon and breast cancer.

With respect to the cereal intake, the results of analytical studies are **inconsistent**, less than a half showed that cereal intake reduced the risk of breast cancer (reviewed in Gerber, 1998; Potishman *et al.*, 1999). The reduction of risk by consumption of cereals is deemed **possible** for stomach cancer and **insufficient** for colon cancer in the WCRF (1997).

Table II. Characteristics and results of recent case-control studies on the fruit and vegetable and cancer relationship

Cancers and pre-cancer conditions	Authors	Country Methodological characteristics	OR	Trend	Remarks
Oro-pharyngeal	Franceschi et al., 1999	Italy case: 598 controls: 1,491	Raw vegetables: H (> 14.1 servings/week) vs L (5 servings/week): 0.4 (0.3-0.6) Cooked vegetables: H (> 4.5 servings/week) vs L (1.5 servings/week): 0.5 (0.3-0.7)	< 0.01 < 0.01	
Stomach	Ji et al., 1998	China cases: 1,124 controls: 1,451	H (≥ 9 servings/day) vs L (6 5) 0.4 (0.3-0.5)	< 0.0001	After sub-groups, only green-yellow vegetables 0.5 (0.4-0.7) T: 0.0001
Lung	Nyberg et al., 1998	Sweden cases: 124 controls: 235	Fruits except citrus H (daily) vs L (2-4/week) 0.49 (0.25-0.94)	0.03	Expressed as a frequency of consumption. Tomatoes: 0.79 (0.43-1.46) T: 0.4
Colo-rectal adenomas	Witte et al., 1996	United States cases: 519 controls: 556	Vegetables H (45.5 servings/week) vs L (9 servings/week) 0.47 (0.29-0.76)	< 0.001	Carotenoid rich vegetables, cruciferous, vitamin C rich fruits significant OR < 1
Colon, rectum	Franceschi et al., 1997	Italy cases: 1,953 controls: 4,154	Vegetables H (> 18.1 servings/week) vs F (8.4) 0.57 (0.47-0.69) Fruits except citrus H (> 19 servings/week) vs L (7.2) 0.72 (0.60-0.87)	< 0.01	Raw vegetables (lettuce, carrots) Cooked green vegetables; peas and beans
Breast	Longnecker et al., 1997	United States cases: 3,543 controls: 9,406	Raw and cooked carrots and spinach H (> 2/week) vs L (< 1/month) 0.56 (0.34-0.91)	0.0001	Each separately less protective No effect of carotene and vit. A supplements
	Favero et al., 1998	Italy cases: 2,569 controls: 2,588	Raw vegetables H (> 12.5 servings/week) vs L (4.9) 0.73 (0.6-0.9)	< 0.01	

H: highest amount; L: lowest amount.

Table III. Characteristics and results of recent prospective studies on the fruit and vegetable and cancer relationship

Cancers and pre-cancer conditions	Authors	Country Methodological characteristics	OR	Trend	Remarks
Stomach	Galanis et al., 1998	Hawaiian Japanese 108/11,907	H ≥ 2/day) vs L (< 1/day) 0.4 (0.2-0.8)	0.02	
	Terry et al., 1998	Sweden 116/11,500	L vs H: 5.5 (1.7-18.3)	< 0.05	
	Botterweck et al., 1998	Netherlands 310/3,500 (sub cohort)	H (374 g/day) vs L (250 g/day) 0.72 (0.48-1.10)	0.14	0.49 (0.20-1.18) cases and pre-cancer conditions vegetables only low variation in intake
Lung	Ocké et al., 1997	Netherlands 19 years; 54/561	Fruits: L (< 107 g/day) vs H (> 166 g/day) 1.92 (1.04-3.55)	0.03	Men: stability of fruit consumption: 2.52 (1.15-5.57). Vegetables: NS
	Knekt et al., 1999	Finland 25 years; 138/4,545	H vs L (non specified) 0.60 (0.38-0.965)	0.02	Fruits 0.58 (0.37-0.93) p: 0.013. Root vegetables 0.56 (0.36-0.88) p: 0.03
Breast	Verhoeven et al., 1997	Netherlands 4 years 650/1,812 (sub-cohort)	Fruits: H (343.1 g/day) vs L (64.9 g/day) 0.76 (0.54-1.08)	0.10	
	Zhang et al., 1999	United States 14 years, 784/83,234	Vegetables H (≥ 5 servings) vs L (< 2 servings) 0.64 (0.43-0.95)	0.10	OR for cancers in pre-menopause
Ovary	Kushi et al., 1999	United States 9 years; 139/29,083	Green leave vegetables: H (> 6 servings/week) vs L (<2) 0.44 (0.25-0.79)	0.01	
Bladder	Michaud et al., 1999	United States 10 years; 252/47,909	H (> 8 servings/day) vs L (< 3.5) 0.72 (0.47-1.09)	0.09	Cruciferous 0.49 (0.32-0.75) T: 0,008

H: highest amount; L: lowest amount.

> **Refined cereals, whole cereals**
>
> A point must be cleared: Italian case-control studies (Favero *et al.*, 1998; Franceschi *et al.*, 1996; Franceschi *et al.*, 1998c) showed that cereal-based foods are a risk factor for colon-rectum and breast cancer. This is not in contradiction with what has just been stated. Today cereal-based products are highly refined. Therefore, they contain little associated nutrients (such as lignans, see further on) and mostly starch. The latter is a major provider of energy which, when in excess, represent a risk for those two types of cancer. When refined and whole cereals are separated, the latter appear inversely associated with the risk of colon, breast and other types of cancers (Franceschi *et al.*, 1998-b; La Vecchia and Chatenoud, 1998; Levi *et al.*, 1999).

Finally, with respect to legumes it should be noted that a case-control study carried out in Majorca (Benito *et al.*, 1990) showed a protective effect of legumes and that Franceschi *et al.*, (1998a) showed that peas and beans reduced the risk of colon cancer.

An attempt was made to identify the nutrients present in these plant foods that could explain this protective effect, sometimes forgetting the difficulty in qualitatively characterising and quantitatively estimating these nutrients in the food composition tables.

Nutrients

Fibres

It should be remembered that the main source of fibres are cereals, legumes and to a lesser extent vegetables and fruits, except for dried fruits.

The beneficial effect of vegetables, especially in cases of intestinal cancer, could be due to the non digestible fraction of plant cell walls: fibres. In the cases of cancer, the beneficial effect of cereal fibres is generally less clear than that of fruit and vegetable fibres, except for whole cereals, which are generally associated with a reduction in the risk of cancers (Jacobs *et al.*, 1995; Vecchia *et al.*, 1998) and in particular colo-rectal cancer (Franceschi *et al.*, 1998b).

Cancer of the colon

Epidemiology
The consensus conference (ECP, 1997) agreed on the strong presumption of protection against colo-rectal cancer by fibres, and it is deemed **possible** by the WRCF (1997).

> In a meta-analysis combining 13 case-control studies, those who ingested the most fibres had about two times less risk of cancer of the colon, than those who ate the least amount (Howe *et al.*, 1992). The analysis by Witte *et al.* (1996) suggested that the risk reducing effect of whole cereals for colo-rectal adenomas is partly due to fibres. However, 4 major prospective studies out of 6 do not demonstrate a relationship between fibres and cancer of the colon, the other two showed a decreased risk in those who consumed the most vegetable fibres. In 2 intervention studies, fibres did not have the expected protective effect: volunteers receiving everyday a wheat germ supplement for 2 years had at least as much development of large adenomas than the controls (McKeow-Essen *et al.*, 1994;

> MacLennan *et al.*, 1995). However, in an Australian study (MacLennan *et al.*, 1995) fibre supplementation increased the risk reduction in the development of large adenomas due to a low in lipid intake.

Mechanisms
Several mechanisms of action of fibres in cancer of the colon are possible:

- increase in faecal volume and in the speed of transit within the intestine, which would decrease the exposure of the colic mucosa to potential carcinogenic compounds in the content;
- decrease in the conversion of primary biliary acids into secondary, probable promoters. Two intervention studies comprising one wheat germ and calcium and the other resistant starch (which is found in the colon like fibres) seem to support the plausibility of this mechanism (Alberts *et al.*, 1996; Hylla *et al.*, 1998);
- production of butyrate, a volatile fatty acid which inhibits *in vitro* the growth of tumour cells and strengthens the immune response (Meflah *et al.*, 1996);
- prevention or reversion of insulin-resistance syndrome that is colon and other (kidney and hormone-dependent cancers) risk factor.

Breast cancer

Epidemiology
Six out of eleven case-control studies (reviewed in Gerber, 1998 and De Stefani *et al.*, 1997) demonstrated a reduction in the risk of breast cancer for the consumption of fibres, with a dose-response effect. The study by Van't Veer *et al.* (1991) in particular showed an interaction between a large intake of fibres and a low intake of fat in the reduction of the risk of breast cancer. Two prospective studies out of four showed only a non-significant decrease in the risk of breast cancer with the consumption of cereals. Therefore, the protective effect is deemed **possible**.

Mechanisms
Fibres act on oestrogen metabolisms according to the following two mechanisms:

- Golding *et al.* (1982) compared levels of plasma oestrogens in vegetarian and omnivorous women. Oestrogen excretion increased when faecal volume increases, and at the same time plasma oestrogen levels decreased. Fibres that increase when volume increases, also adsorb oestrogens whose promoter effect on breast cancer cells is known. It was observed that the faecal oestrogen level increased with an acceleration in intestinal transit (Lewis *et al.*, 1997).
- Fibres allow the multiplication of β-glycuronidase free bacteria. For this reason, oestrogens escape from bacterial deconjugation and from entero-hepatic recycling (reviewed in Gerber, 1996a; and Gerber, 1998).

Whatever the mechanism, several studies have demonstrated that a fibre supplementation (combined with a low lipid diet) in non-menopausal volunteers significantly decreased the concentrations of serum oestradiol and oestrone (reviewed in Gerber, 1998). Given the promotional effect of oestrogens on breast cancer cells, their decrease in serum could explain a reduction of the risk.

Phyto-oestrogens
These compounds have two plant-origin precursors, isoflavones and lignans. These are transformed by the colon flora into equol and enterodiol and enterolactone, respectively, whose structure is similar to that of oestrogens and are capable of binding the β receptor of oestrogens. Isoflavonoids are found in legumes, especially in soybean, but also in Mediterranean legumes: lentils, beans, and chickpeas. Lignan sources are principally sesame seeds, unrefined cereals and perhaps also cruciferous plants, and vegetables and fruits rich in carotenoids (Wiseman, 1999).

Epidemiology
The interaction of phyto-oestrogens with hormone metabolism was initially observed in animals, sheep grazing in clover fields became sterile thus revealing the anti-oestrogenic effect of these compounds. In women, small nutritional interventions with soybean proteins (Cassidy *et al.*, 1994) and soybean milk (Nagata *et al.*, 1998) demonstrated that such diets tended to decrease the level of certain oestrogens and/or lengthen the menstrual cycle, which results in a lower oestrogenic impregnation over the entire life. It was also observed that Japanese women who consumed large amounts of soy-bean presented less breast cancer than women with an occidental type diet. Finally, a study carried out in Australia showed that a high isoflavonoid phyto-oestrogen urinary level was associated with a reduced risk of breast cancer (Ingram *et al.*, 1997). For the other hormone-dependent cancers the studies are more rare, however a protective effect of the consumption of soybean and other sources of phyto-oestrogens have been reported for cancer of the endometrium (Goodmann *et al.*, 1997).

Mechanisms
Phyto-oestrogens seem to modify hormone metabolism by the structural similarity with human oestrogens.

Possible interaction of phyto-oestrogens with hormone metabolism

Phyto-oestrogens bind the β receptor of oestrogens, on which they have a slight agonist effect, thus inducing light oestrogen synthesis. The β receptor is the one that is distributed over all the tissues which benefit from oestrogen replacement therapy (bone, brain and cardiovascular tissue). This cell biology observation was related to the descriptive epidemiological studies reporting that the symptoms related to a drop in oestrogen levels during menopause are virtually absent in Japanese women. Soybean consumption provides a major source of phyto-oestrogens in the diet of the latter: therefore soybean phyto-oestrogens behave as agonists on the tissues with the β receptor.
However, phyto-oestrogens have a lower affinity for oestrogen α receptors, which are the majority in normal or tumour breast tissue. In this case, phyto-oestrogens behave as negative modulators of the α receptor and therefore present an antagonist effect. However, according to some authors, some effects of phyto-oestrogens do not take place *via* the receptors but *via* intracellular signalling effects.

Anti-oxidants
Given that anti-oxidant nutrients β-carotene, vitamins C and E are present in many plant products with a proven protective role, these nutrients were automatically associated with this protective effect when the foods were transformed in nutrients, even though it was not possible to define if they were responsible for the risk reduction or just markers of fruit and vegetable consumption, which are protectors *via* other possible components.

Epidemiology
Beta-carotenes and other carotenoids
Studies on the food intake or the plasma levels of _-carotene showed **convincing** protective results with respect to cancer of the oesophagus, lung and stomach cancer. Results are **consistent but limited** for cancer of the larynx and of the uterus and **insufficient** for oro-pharyngeal cancer and of the pancreas. The effects are **consistent or insufficient** for all the other cancers *(Tables IV to VII)*.

Contrary to the apparently protective role of tomatoes (see above), the results of various studies concerning lycopene, the main tomato carotenoid, seem to be disappointing except for prostate cancer, whose risk was decreased in the study by a high lycopene intake (Giovanucci et al., 1995) and in another by a high lycopene plasma level (Gann et al., 1999), however it is difficult to reach a conclusion due to the small number of studies, the insufficiency of the food composition tables, and for the studies based on plasma levels, due to the difficulty in interpreting the levels observed (lycopene does not remain for long in plasma and is not a good food marker).

When its effect was tested directly on humans in intervention trials *(Table I)*, β-carotene did not show a protective effect, but on the contrary it increased significantly the risk of lung cancer in Finnish smokers (+ 18%) (ATBC, 1994) and also in the CARET study (Omenn et al., 1996). More recently an intervention trial comparing the effect of vitamin A to that of β-carotene (without placebo group) in workers exposed to asbestos showed that vitamin A reduced the risk relative to β-carotene and that the number of mesotheliomas in the β-carotene treated group was greater than expected (de Klerk et al., 1998).

For colon cancer, β-carotene supplementation seems also to increase the recurrence of colon adenomas in two intervention studies but the OR is not significant (Greenberg et al., 1994; MacLennan et al., 1995).

However the latest Italian results (table IV) continue to demonstrate a risk reducing effect of β-carotene (La Vecchia et al., 1997). The same group also showed a reducing effect for β-carotene on thyroid cancer (d'Avanzo et al., 1997) and for breast cancer in 2,569 cases and 2,588 controls (La Vecchia et al., 1998). After close analysis of this study (Mezzeti et al., 1998), a low β-carotene level (< 3.4 mg per day) would explain 15% of breast cancers. However, for the latter cancer, most of studies showed negative results (reviewed in IARC, 1998) as were the last major studies carried out in Northern Europe EURAMIC and the Netherlands Cohort Study (Van't Veer et al., 1996; Verhoeven et al., 1997). A recent prospective study carried out in the United States suggested a protective effect for lycopene, β-cryptoxanthine and luteine/zeaxanthine even though the OR are not significant (Dorgan et al., 1998). However, since it has been mentioned that there is a possibility of the presence of lignans in carotenoid rich foods, it could be thought that at the high consumption levels observed in Mediterranean countries (> 4 mg per day), these vegetables provide enough lignans to play their protective role.

Table IV. Carotenoids and cancers. Recent case-control studies based on consumption

Cancers and pre-cancer conditions	Authors	Country Methodological characteristics	OR	Trend	Remarks
Salivary gland	Horn-Ross et al., 1997	United States cases: 133 controls: 191	carotene H (> 3.9 mg/day) vs L (≤ 2.1 mg/day) 0.54 (0.2-0.99)	0.05	Becomes NS after adjustment for vitamin C
Stomach	Ji et al., 1998	China cases: 1,124 controls: 1,451	carotene Men: H (≥ 1.5 g/day) vs L (≤ 0.74 g/day) 0.4 (0.3-0.6) Women: H (1.3 g/day) vs L (0.66 g/day) 0.7 (0.5-1.1)	Men < 0.0001 Women: 0,02	Adjustment for alcohol and tobacco only in men
	Kaaks et al., 1998	Belgium cases: 301 controls: 2,851	β-carotene H vs L (non specified) 0.50 p < 0.05	< 0.001	
	Garcia-Closas et al., 1999	Spain cases: 354 controls: 354	Carotenoids H vs L (mg/day): β-carotene < 0.6 vs > 2.9 α-carotene <0.02 vs 0.2; luteine < 0.3 vs > 1. all NS	NS	Kaempferol protector 0.48 (0.26-0.88) T: 0.04
Colon, rectum	La Vecchia et al., 1997	Italy cases: 1,953 controls: 4,154	Carotenoids H (= 7.7 mg/day) vs L (3.6-4.9 mg/day) 0.63 (0.5-0.8)	< 0.001	Continuous OR: 0.87 (0.8-1.0)
	Ghadirian et al., 1997	Canada cases: 402 controls: 668	β-carotene H vs L (non specified) 0.72 (0.49-1.06)	–	
Breast	Negri et al., 1996-a	Italy cases: 2,569 controls: 2,588	β-carotene H (> 5.8 mg/day) vs L (= 2.8 mg/day) 0.74 (0.6-0.9)	< 0.01	Mutual adjustment on other micronutrients: 0.84 (0.7-1.0) T < 0.05
	La Vecchia et al., 1998	Italy cases: 2,569 controls: 2,588 same study as above	β-carotene H (= 6.6 mg/day) vs L (< 3.0 mg/day) 0.68 (0.56-0.82) α-carotene H (> 1.2 mg/day) vs L (< 0.3 mg/day) 0.58 (0.48-0.70)	< 0.001	
	Bohlke et al., 1999	Greece cases: 820 controls: 1,548	β-carotene H (> 8.3 mg/day) vs L (3.8 mg/day) 0.67 (0.49- 0.91)	0.005	preM: 0.36 (0.21-0.61) T: 0.0001 postM: NS
Endometrium	Negri et al., 1996-b	Italy cases: 368 controls: 713	β-carotene H (> 5.5 mg/day) vs L (2.9 mg/day) 0.5	< 0.01	IC not given questionnaire of 50 foods
Prostate	Key et al., 1997	Great Britain cases: 328 controls: 328	carotene H (= 3.48 mg/day) vs L (< 2.65 mg/day) 0.83 (0.57-1.21)	NS	
Thyroid	d'Avanzo et al., 1997	Italy cases: 399 controls: 617	β-carotene H (= 5.8 mg/day) vs L (< 3.1 mg/day) 0.58 (0.4-0.9)	< 0.05	Questionnaire of 29 foods

H: highest amount; L: lowest amount; NS: non significant.

Table V. Carotenoids and cancers. Recent case-control studies based on tissue levels

Cancers and pre-cancer conditions	Authors	Country Methodological characteristics	OR	Trend	Remarks
Colorectal polyps	Shikany et al., 1997	United States cases: 472 controls: 502	β-carotene in plasma (μmol/1) H (> 0.486) vs L (< 0.186) OR= 1.05 (0.712-1.57)	NS	All carotenoids NS after adjustment on fruits and vegetables
Breast	van't Veer et al., 1996	5 European countries post-menopause cases: 347 controls: 374	β-carotene, adipose tissue H (1.33 μg/g) vs L (0.69) OR: 0.74 (0.45-1.23)	NS	Euramic Study No interaction No effect of anti-oxidant composite score
	Zhang et al., 1997	United States cases: 46 controls: 63	β-carotene, mammary fat H (> median, non specified) vs L (< median) OR: 0.30 (0.11-0.85)	–	Different samples collected at an interval of one year No correlation to intake

H: highest amount; L: lowest amount; NS: non significant.

Vitamin C
A reduction in risk due to vitamin C consumption is **convincing** for stomach cancer, **probable** for oro-pharyngeal, larynx, lung and bronchi, pancreas and cervix cancers. Results are insufficient for all other types of cancer *(Tables VIII and IX)*.

There are few intervention studies with vitamin C. The Linxian study (Blot, 1993) included a group supplemented with this vitamin (plus molybdenum) but did not show any effect.

Vitamin E
Vitamin E supplementation seems to give **inconsistent** results for lung and upper respiratory tract cancers *(Tables X to XIII)* while a protection was demonstrated against prostate cancer (Heinoen *et al.*, 1998). Two prospective studies based on vitamin E serum levels (Eichholzer *et al.*, 1992; Gann *et al.*, 1999, *Table XIII*) showed that aggressive prostate tumours (*i.e.* rapid evolution) are associated with low vitamin E levels in smokers. The number of cases is small, but like for lycopene it is a research that must be continued.

Breast and colon cancer did **not show any association** with vitamin E.

Other anti-oxidants
As seen before, plants also provide consumers with micronutrients that are neither vitamins nor nutrients, but that seem to be for the most part beneficial. However, few studies have been able to study this aspect given the absence of full and reliable data on food composition. The best known are the phenolic compounds, including flavonols and flavanols. Hertog *et al.* (1993) did not find any flavonol effect on cancer mortality. Studying the incidence of

Table VI. Carotenoids and cancers. Recent prospective studies based on consumption

Cancers and pre-cancer conditions	Authors	Country Methodological characteristics	OR	Trend	Remarks
Lung	Ocké et al., 1997	Netherlands prospective (19) 54/561 men	≤ 33th vs > 33th percentile stable intake β-carotene 2.11 (1.02-4.38)	-	NS for the entire sample
	Yong et al., 1997	United States prospective (19) 248/10,068	Carotenoids H (2,290 IU) vs L (< 206.2 IU) 0.74 (0.52-1.06)	0.14	+ vit. C + E. 0.32 (0.14-0.74): T:0.0004; +vit.C: 0.41 (0.24-0.72) T: 0.0003; + vit. E 0.62 (0.36-1.08) T: 0.04
	Knekt et al., 1999	Finland prospective (25) 138/4,545	β-carotene H (non specified) vs L (26 µg/day) 0.61 (0.39-0.95)	0.10	β-carotene NS Smokers vs non-smokers NS. Lycopene without effect
Breast	Kushi et al., 1996	United States, postM prospective (6) 879/34,387	Carotenoids ingested H vs L (non specified) 0.88 (0.70-1.12)	NS	OR = 1 in women not supplemented with vitamins A, C and E
	Verhoeven et al., 1997	Netherlands prospective (4,3) 650/1,812 (subcohort)	β-carotene (mg/day H-0.7 vs L-0.2) 1.01 (0.72-1.42)	NS	
	Zhang et al., 1999	United States 2,697/83,234 (18 years)	β-carotene (mg/day H-7.6 vs F-1.7) α-carotene (1.5 vs 0.2) for both OR 0.84 (0.67-1.05) β-cryptoxanthine (0.7 vs 0.02) 0.89 (0.70-1.13) luteine/zea (8.8 vs 1.4) 0.79 (0.63-0.99)	NS NS NS 0,04	Cases in pre-menopause only Effect in post-menopause when HRT and in women with family history of breast cancer

H: highest amount; L: lowest amount; NS: non significant.

Table VII. Carotenoids and cancers. Recent prospective studies based on plasma concentrations

Cancers and pre-cancer conditions	Authors	Country Methodological characteristics	OR	Trend	Remarks
Stomach	Eichholzer et al., 1996	Switzerland (17) 24/2974	Carotene L (< 0.23 µm/1) vs H (≥ 0.23 µm/1) 3.30 (1.42-7.70)		Continuous covariables, first 2 years of follow-up excluded
Lung	Eichholzer et al., 1996	Switzerland (17) 87/2974	Carotene L (< 0.23 µm/1) vs H (≥ 0.23 µm/1) 1.90 (1.18-3.07)		Continuous covariables, first 2 years of follow-up excluded
	Comstock et al., 1997	United States blood donors (8 years) cases: 258 selection of paired controls 515	Carotenoids (H vs L, not defined) carotene: 0.44 β-carotene: 0.48 cryptoxanthine: 0.2 luteinee/zeaxanthine: 0.41	0.002 0.01 < 0.001 < 0.001	
Colon, rectum	Eichholzer et al., 1996	Switzerland (17) 21/2974	Carotene L (< 0.23 µm/l) vs H (= 0.23 µm/l) 1.33 (0.47-3.80)		Continuous covariables, first 2 years of follow-up excluded
Prostate	Eichholzer et al., 1996	Switzerland (17) 29/2974	β-carotene L (< 0.23 µm/l) vs H (= 0.23 µm/l) 1.03 (0.43-2.47)		Continuous covariables, first 2 years of follow-up excluded
	Gann et al., 1999	United States Physicians Health Study cases: 578 paired controls: 1,294	0.57 (0.37-0.88) in subjects with L level of lycopene	NS	
Breast	Dorgan et al., 1998	United States (9.5) 105/7,224	β-carotene H (0.69-2.20 µm/1) vs F (= 0.29 µm/1) 1.1 (0.5-2.4)	NS	

H: highest amount; L: lowest amount; NS: non significant.

Table VIII. Vitamin C and cancers. Recent prospective studies based on consumption

Cancers and pre-cancer conditions	Authors	Country Methodological characteristics	OR	Trend	Remarks
Lung	Ocké et al., 1997	Netherlands Men follow-up: 19 years 54/561	L (< 80 mg/day) vs H (> 102 mg/day) 2.16 (1.14-4.09)	0.02	
	Yong et al., 1997	United States follow-up: 19 years 248/10,068	H (> 113.055 mg/day) vs F < 23.07 mg/day) 0.66 (0.45-0.96)	0.01	+ vit. E + carot. 0.32 (0.14-0.74) T: 0.0004 + vit. E: 0.40 (0.20-0.80) T: 0.0003; + carot: 0.41 (0.24-0.72) T: 0.04
Breast	Kushi et al., 1996	United States follow-up: 6 years 879/34,387 post-menopause	H (≥ 392 mg/day) vs L (< 112 mg/day) 0.87 (0.70-1.08)	0.88	OR = 1 in women not supplemented with vitamins A, C and E
	Verhoeven et al., 1997	Netherlands follow-up: 4 years 650/1,812 (sub-cohort)	H (165,3 mg/day) vs L (58.6 mg/day) 0.77 (0.55-1.08)	0.08	

H: highest amount; L: lowest amount; NS: non significant.

Table IX. Vitamin C and cancers. Recent prospective studies based on tissue concentrations

Cancers and pre-cancer conditions	Authors	Country Methodological characteristics	OR	Trend	Remarks
Stomach	Eichholzer et al., 1996	Switzerland follow-up: 17 years 24/2,974	plasma conc. L (< 22.7 µm/1) vs H (> 22.7 µm/l) 0.97 (0.44-2.14)	–	
Lung	Eichholzer et al., 1996	Switzerland follow-up: 17 years 87/2,974	plasma conc. L (< 22.7 µm/1) vs H (≥ 22.7 µm/l) 1.82 (0.86-3.85)	–	Associated with low vitamin E levels: 3.70 (1.61-8.52)
Colon	Eichholzer et al., 1996	Switzerland follow-up: 17 years 21/2,974	plasma conc. L (< 22.7 µm/1) vs H (> 22.7 µm/l) L vs H 0.90 (0.34-2.34)	–	

H: highest amount; L: lowest amount; NS: non significant.

Table X. Vitamin E and cancers. Recent case-control studies based on consumption

Cancers and pre-cancer conditions	Authors	Country Methodological characteristics	OR	Trend	Remarks
Salivary gland	Horn-Ross et al., 1997	United States cases: 133 controls: 184	H (> 14 mg/day) vs L (≤ 7 mg/day) 0.69 (0.38-1.2)	0.22	Becomes 1.2 (0.58-2.3) after adjusting for vitamin C
Stomach	Ji et al., 1998	China cases: 1,124 controls: 1,451	Men: H (≥ 31.7 mg/day) vs L (≤ 19.7 mg/day) 0.5 (0.3-0.7) Women: H (≥ 28.8 mg/day) vs L (≤ 17.2 mg/day) 0.5 (0.31-0.8)	Men: < 0.0001 Women: 0.0002	Adjustment for alcohol and smoking in men only
Colon, rectum	La Vecchia et al., 1997	Italy cases: 1,953 controls: 4,154	H (≥ 18.42 mg/day) vs L (9.72-12.31) 0.45 (0.4-0.6)	< 0.001	Continuous OR: 0.65 (0.6-0.7)
	Ghadirian et al., 1997	Canada cases: 402 controls: 668	H vs L (undefined) 0.53 (0.26-0.78)	–	α-tocopherol (supplements) 0.63 (0.43-0.94)
Breast	Negri et al., 1996-a	Italy cases: 2,569 controls: 2,588	H (> 13.43 mg/day) vs L (≤ 7.21 mg/day) 0.69 (0.6-0.8)	< 0.01	continuous OR 0.84 (0.78-0.91) continuous mutual adjustment: 0.86 (0.79-0.94)
	Bohlke et al., 1999	Greece cases: 820 controls: 1,548	H (> 8.6 IU/day) vs L (≤ 5.2 IU/day) 0.71 (0.48-1.05)	0.04	preM: 0.50 (0.25-1.02) tend: 0.03; postM: NS after mutual adjustment
Thyroid	d'Avanzo et al., 1997	Italy cases: 399 controls: 617	H (≥ 15 mg/day) vs F (< 9 mg/day) 0.67 (0.4-1)	NS	29 foods

H: highest amount; L: lowest amount; NS: non significant.

Table XI. Vitamin E and cancers. Recent case-control studies based on adipose tissue concentrations

Cancers and pre-cancer conditions	Authors	Country Methodological characteristics	OR	Trend	Remarks
Breast	van'tVeer et al., 1996	Europe postM cases: 347 controls: 374	adipose tissue H (350 mg/g) vs L (231 mg/g) 1.15 (0.75-1.77)	0.31	Euramic: 5 centres, antioxidants composite score 1.54 (0.94-2.52)

H: highest amount; L: lowest amount; NS: non significant.

Table XII. Vitamin E and cancers. Recent prospective studies based on consumption

Cancers and pre-cancer conditions	Authors	Country Methodological characteristics	OR	Trend	Remarks
Lung	Ocké et al., 1997	Netherlands Men follow-up: 19 years 54/561	F (< 15.3 mg/day) vs L (> 19.8 mg/day) 1.47 (0.66-3.17)	NS	
	Yong et al., 1997	United States follow-up: 19 years 248/10,068	H (> 6.71 mg/day) vs L (< 3.69 mg/day) 0.88 (0.62-1.25)	NS	+ vit. C + carot. 0.32 (0.14-0.74) T: 0.0004 + vit C: 0.40 (0.20-0.80) T: 0.0003; + carot: 0.62 (0.36-1.,08) T: 004
Breast	Kushi et al., 1996	United States post-M follow-up: 6 years 879/34,387	H (≥ 35.66 mg/day) vs L (< 5.66 mg/day) 1.05 (0.83-1.33)	NS	Id. in women not supplemented with vitamins A, C and E
	Verhoeven et al., 1997	Netherlands follow-up: 4 years 650/1,812 (sub-cohort)	H (19.82 mg/day) vs L (5.96 mg/day) 1.25 (0.85-1.85)	NS	

H: highest amount; L: lowest amount; NS: non significant.

various cancers in a Finnish cohort, Knekt *et al.* (1997) demonstrated a significantly protective effect of flavonols on lung cancer. Therefore results are limited.

Mechanisms
Anti-oxidants are capable of protecting DNA against oxidative stress, but they can also inhibit the synthesis of growth factors by acting on transmembrane signals. Carotenoids can play this role (IARC, 1998) as well as vitamin E, especially when combined with vitamin C (Gerber, 1996b). Flavonols such as quercetin and kaempferol, have anti-oxidant properties; it has been demonstrated that the efficacy of flavonoids in protecting DNA from oxidative stress depends on the number and position of hydroxyl radicals (Noroozi *et al.*, 1998). This anti-oxidant capacity can also explain their inhibitory effect on proliferation (Fotsi *et al.*, 1997). However, daidzein and genistein can also block the cell cycle and thus inhibit proliferation. Garlic and onion sulphur compounds (diallyl sulphide) and other phenolic compounds (caffeic acid) may also present an anti-oxidant capacity, and also act as a modulator of phase I and phase II enzymes, as well as glucosinolates, isothiocyanates, and terpenes whose role in cancerogenesis is known (*see also technical information:* "Polyphenols: an introduction").

Table XIII. Vitamin E and cancers. Recent prospective studies based on plasma concentrations

Cancers and pre-cancer conditions	Authors	Country Methodological characteristics	OR	Trend	Remarks
Stomach	Eichholzer et al., 1996	Switzerland follow-up: 17 years 24/2,974	F (< 30.02 µm/l) vs H (> 30.02 µm/l) 0.52 (0.20-1.34)		
Lung	Eichholzer et al., 1996	Switzerland follow-up: 17 years 83/2,974	F (< 30.02 µm/l) vs H (> 30.02 µm/l) 1.03 (0.60-1.78)		Associated with low vitamin C levels: 3.76 (1.63-8.71)
Colon	Eichholzer et al., 1996	Switzerland follow-up: 17 years 21/2,974	F (< 30.02 µm/l) vs H (> 30.02 µm/l) 1.33 (0.47-3.80)		
Prostate	Eichholzer et al., 1996	Switzerland follow-up: 17 years 29/2,974	F (< 30.02 µm/l) vs H (> 30.02 µm/l) smokers: 19.89 (3.6-109.8) non smokers: 5.66 (0.88-36.34)		Cases observed during the first 2 years of follow-up excluded: 8.34 (1.01-68.7) 3.07 (0.55-17.3)
	Gann et al., 1999	United States Physicians Health Study cases: 578 paired controls: 1,294	H (> 33.5) vs L (< 19.9) 1.06 (0.76-1.48)	NS	Aggressive cases only (259) 0.64 (0.38-1.07) T: 0.11 aggressive cases in smokers + ex-smokers: 0.51 (0.26-0.98)

H: highest amount; L: lowest amount; NS: non significant.

How to explain the results difference between the observations concerning fruit and vegetables and those concerning nutrients?

It was thought that the protective effect of fruit and vegetables came from the combination of several factors and not from a single molecule. The study of Yong et al. (1997) on lung cancers strongly suggests this *(Tables VI, VIII and XII)*.

Intervention studies have tried this protocol as a "cocktail". Volunteers who received every day a β-carotene and vitamins C and E supplements for 2 to 4 years had equal recurrence of adenomatous polyps as controls (McKeown-Eyssen et al., 1998; De Cosse et al., 1989; Greenberg et al., 1994). Therefore, apparently the appearance and/or growth of colon tumours cannot be prevented by these anti-oxidants. In a malnourished rural China population, β-carotene and vitamin E, combined with selenium (cofactor of glutathion-peroxidase, anti-oxidant enzyme) administered for 5 years decreased mortality for all cancers and for stomach cancer (Blot et al., 1993). The same study did not demonstrate any protection against stomach cancer by supplements of vitamin C combined with molybdenum. However, as we have seen, many micro-components of fruit and vegetables are badly identified on the one hand, badly evaluated on the other hand, and finally it is still difficult to evaluate the synergy mechanisms among the different plant components.

> **How to explain the failure of intervention studies by β-carotene and to a lesser extent vitamin E supplementation?**
>
> It could be that the follow-up is not long enough to show results, or that β-carotene is not a protective element in fruit and vegetable. Apart from phenolic compounds, the components of certain Mediterranean foods, such as allyl sulphides in garlic and onion, glucosinolates, isothiocyanates and terpenes in citrus fruits could be anti-carcinogens as demonstrated by *in vitro* animal experiments. However, this confusion in the cause does not explain the risk increase with β-carotene supplementation. It seems that there remain too many non elucidated elements relative to the dose and possible and/or necessary combinations to supplement in a nutrient basis. There are also too many gaps relative to the natural history of cancer, and this is surely best illustrated by the results of the ATBC and CARET studies which had both recruited subjects already presenting a transformation of bronchial and pulmonary epithelium cells into cancer cells. Under these conditions, and in the possible presence of a persistent oxidative stress (smoking) anti-oxidants could have acted as pro-oxidants, and/or favour cell proliferation by protecting it from oxidative stress (Gerber, 1996b; Gerber *et al.*, 1996a; Gerber *et al.*, 1997; Saintot *et al.*, 1997; IARC, 1998).

Other diseases

A certain number of other pathologies could benefit from the Mediterranean diet: age-related macular degeneration, cataracts and cognitive ageing for which a risk reduction has been related to a major intake of anti-oxidants. Also, it has been demonstrated that an anti-oxidant supplementation improves pulmonary ventilation of subjects living (Romieu *et al.*, 1998) or practising a physical activity (Girevink *et al.*, 1998; Grievink *et al.*, 1999) in ozone contaminated environments. With respect to folates, it is known that an intake greater than 400 μg per day in pregnant women decreases the risk of spina bifida. However no study has examined the difference in incidence or morbidity of this disease between Mediterranean countries and other countries that would allow the suggestion of a benefit specifically linked to the Mediterranean diet.

Low meat consumption, mainly lamb and goat

Cardiovascular diseases

Epidemiology

A major characteristic of Mediterranean diets is the very low proportion of red meat (approximately 3 times less than in Northern European countries). It seems that a large consumption of red meat is associated with several chronic pathologies. Practically all the studies carried out with vegetarians showed that they have a distinctly lower risk of cardiac incident than non-vegetarians (reviewed in Corpet and Gerber, 1997). However, the influence of confusion factors, such as physical activity and smoking, cannot be excluded from these studies.

Mechanisms

How can red meat influence cardiovascular diseases? In general the harmful effects of meat are attributed to their cholesterol and saturated fat content. These nutrients clearly influence cholesterolemia, a major risk factor of cardiovascular diseases. Indeed, when red meat is added for several days to a vegetarian diet, LDL cholesterol increases as well as systolic blood pressure (Sachs *et al.* 1981)

Haeme iron, for which red meat is the major source, also seems associated to cardiovascular diseases. In a Finnish study, the risk of infarction was associated with iron reserves (serum ferritin, Salonen *et al.*, 1992), which are themselves dependent on haeme iron intake that is better absorbed than non-haeme iron. In a prospective study (Ascherio *et al.*, 1994), haeme iron was associated to the risk while non-haeme iron, provided mainly by vegetables, was not related. In their 1997 review, Corti *et al.* thought that the results were inconsistent, however a recent study carried out in Greece demonstrated an increased risk in cardiovascular diseases associated to iron intake: for a monthly increase of 50 mg/month in iron consumption, the OR increases to 1.47 (IC: 1.02-1.12) for men and 3.61 (IC: 1.45-9.01) for women (Tzonou *et al.*, 1998). Iron can trigger the generation of free radicals (Fenton's reaction).

Cancers

Cancer of the colon

Epidemiology

The review by Potter *et al.* (1993) showed that in 16 analytical studies out of 27, the consumption of red meat is associated with an increased risk of cancer of the colon. Potter concluded that if the studies that were not well conducted were excluded, more than 8 out of 10 studies showed a risk associated with the consumption of red meat. The two large prospective studies carried out in the United States clearly show the risk associated to red meat consumption, while on the contrary the consumption of poultry and fish was associated with a reduction in risk (Willet *et al.*, 1990; Giovannucci *et al.*, 1994). Another prospective study, carried out in Sweden, also showed the link between beef or lamb consumption and the risk (Gerhardson de Verdier *et al.*, 1991). In a study performed in the Netherlands, the risk of cancer of the colon was only associated with processed meat, cold cuts (Goldbohm *et al.*, 1994). This effect of processed meats is found again in a Norwegian study, with a relative risk of 2.5 in those who eat cold cuts twice a day or more, relative to those who eat less. Finally, 4 other prospective studies, including a recent Hsing *et al.* (1998), are compatible with the hypothesis of a positive association, without finding a significant risk associated with red meat consumption, indicating a **possible** risk.

Mechanisms

It was thought for a long time that the fat in the red meat were the cancer risk factors. A major hypothesis is that fats are the food source with the highest energy concentration, and that an excess of energy would promote numerous cancers. For cancer of the colon, fats favour the production of billiary acids that serve to emulsion them during digestion. Primary billiary acids, after transformation into secondary billiary acids by intestinal bacteria could be promoters of intestinal cancers.

Giovannucci and Goldin (1997) argued against the thesis according to which meat would be a risk factor due to the lipids. On the contrary they support the explanation related to the presence of heterocyclic aromatic amines, which are potential carcinogens, in meat cooked at high temperature (roasted, fried or grilled). Some studies indicate that the risk is more specifically related to the consumption of meat cooked that way. This has been observed for cancer of the colon in certain studies but not in all (Gherardsson de Verdier, 1991).

Breast cancer

Epidemiology
The link between breast cancer and red meat consumption is certainly more controversial than for cancer of the colon.

> A positive association was found with red meat (Toniolo et al., 1989) and also with animal fats (saturated and mono-unsaturated) in various studies, case-control or cohort (Howe et al., 1991; Richardson et al., 1991; Knekt et al., 1990; Kushi et al., 1992; Yu et al., 1990). However, the statistical adjustment models for energy, which try to demonstrate the specific effect of fatty acids, indicate that there is no significant effect (Van den Brandt et al., 1993; Willet et al., 1992; Kushi et al., 1992).

Mechanisms
It has also been thought that fats could be the nutrient in cause. The role of lipids in breast cancer, found in certain studies, could be due to the constitution of excess weight. There would be either synthesis of oestrogens in adipose tissue, and or in case of abdominal type obesity (apple shape), the existence of an insulin-resistance syndrome, which is accompanied by the synthesis of growth factors and a modification of hormone metabolism favouring the promotion and growth of breast tumours (Stoll, 1997 and paragraph 1). The presence of heterocyclic aromatic amines in meat cooked at high temperature has also been reported as a risk factor for breast cancer (Knekt et al., 1994). This mechanism involves the participation of enzymes metabolising xenobiotics, certain genetic polymorphisms confering a greater susceptibility to carcinogenesis (Ambrosone et al., 1997).

> **Genetic polymorphism and cancer**
>
> Proteins, and in particular enzymes, can present variable amino acid sequences (polymorphism), which confer on them variable properties. When this applies to phase I and II enzymes, certain polymorphisms will increase or decrease the activation or detoxification capacity of these enzymes. Thus, the subjects presenting these polymorphisms will have a greater or lesser susceptibility to carcinogens (smoking, heterocyclic aromatic amines, etc.).

Prostate cancer
A review of 9 case-control studies strongly suggests a positive association between red meat consumption and prostate cancer (Nomura et al., 1991). Prospective studies on prostate cancer show a greater risk in those who eat more meat in Hawaii and in the United States, among

health professionals as well as in Adventists (Giovannucci et al., 1993; Le Marchand et al., 1994; Mills et al., 1989). The relative risks associated with meat consumption are significant but not very large. Thus, Adventists who consumed meat every day had a relative risk of cancer of 1.4 relative to non-consumers.

Some fatty acids have been specifically associated with prostate cancer: Giovannucci et al. (1993) and Gann et al. (1994) have demonstrated in two different cohorts (but both North American) and with different methods for evaluating intake, that α-linolenic acid was significantly associated with an increase in risk. This result has been confirmed in the study by Harvei et al. (1997). Normally this is a plant compound; however, in the United States, it may be a confusion factor in meat consumption, as animals for slaughter are often fed with soy cakes, which may contain α-linolenic acid.

As has been described for cardiovascular diseases *(see above)*, red meat provides lots of iron to the body in an easily assimilated form (haeme iron). This metal, required for life, can increase the peroxidation of lipids and the production of free radicals, involved in carcinogenesis.

Finally, and perhaps mainly, meat rich diets are in general low in plant products, and therefore provide fewer protective factors to the consumer.

High fish consumption

Cardiovascular diseases

Epidemiology

It should be noted that the low meat consumption in Mediterranean diet is compensated by a major intake of fish and other sea foods. Now, it has been reported that Eskimos who have a high n-3 fatty acid intake presented fewer cardiovascular diseases (Kromhout et al., 1985). More recently in the United States, an inverse relationship between fish consumption (35 g/day) and myocardial infarction mortality was demonstrated, the mortality was even lower if the "non-sudden" mortality is considered (Daviglus et al., 1997). An anti-fibrillation effect was even shown (Landmark et al., 1998). A recent review (Marckmann and Gronbaek, 1999) mentioned that it is only in the at risk population (for example a high saturated fat intake) that a risk reduction associated with daily fish consumption of more than 30 g is demonstrated.

Mechanisms

It is known that the n-3 series fatty acids, contained in large amounts in fish, improve the lipid parameters which are markers for cardiovascular disease: they decrease triglyceridemia, even with an intake of 40% in lipid calories; they decrease LDL cholesterol without decrease of HDL, in a diet with a 30% lipid intake (Mori et al., 1994). Furthermore, it has been demonstrated in a metabolic study with 50 subjects that daily consumption of 12 g of fish oil combined with 900 mg of garlic decreased both the lipid parameters, total cholesterol and LDL cholesterol, and triglycerides (Adler and Houb, 1997). Cold sea fish generally contain more of these fatty acids, however tuna, sardines and mackerel consumed in Mediterranean countries present levels similar to those of herring and salmon (*see chapter* "Fish and sea foods").

Cancers

Epidemiology
The consumption of fish oils, containing n-3 series fatty acids, EPA and DHA, seem to induce a reduction in the risk of cancer mortality, as suggested by the low cancer mortality in Eskimos (Kaiser *et al.*, 1989). Indeed, these fatty acids are found mainly in cold sea fish. Other studies support this hypothesis (reviewed in Gerber and Corpet, 1997). Three cohort studies out of 6, and 7 case-control studies (reviewed in Giovannuci and Goldin, 1997) showed an inverse association between fish consumption and cancer of the colon. For breast cancer, the same result is obtained in Italy (Favero *et al.*, 1998). Thus, the Mediterranean fatty fish (sardines, mackerels, tuna) could have enough n-3 fatty acids to play a role in cancer prevention.

Mechanisms
It has been demonstrated in animals that these fatty acids inhibit tumour growth in animal models of mammary and colon tumours (reviewed in Bougnoux *et al.*, 1996). It is a substrate competition that results in a decrease in the synthesis of arachidonic acid, therefore of prostaglandins involved in the tumour progression and metastasis process, or a toxic effect on the proliferation of tumour cells.

However, it cannot be overlooked that the mere replacement of meat by fish may induce a reduction in the risk.

No milk or butter, yoghurt and cheese instead

Cardiovascular diseases

Epidemiology
In the so-called "Seven Countries" international study (Keys, 1986), the Finns are those who consume the most milk products, and are also the ones with the highest incidence of cardiovascular accidents. Practically no retrospective or prospective analytical study has been published on the link between milk product consumption and cardiovascular diseases.

Mechanisms
Milk fat contains more saturated fatty acids than the other animal fats (60 to 70% compared to 40 to 50% in beef fat). Furthermore, the saturated medium chain fatty acids found in milk, result in a greater increase in LDL cholesterol, associated to the risk, than the longer chain fatty acids found in beef (Artaud-Wild *et al.*, 1993). Furthermore, it is not known whether saturated fats have the same effect in yoghurt or cheese, for which the milk is first fermented, than in fresh milk products. α-linolenic acid (18:3 n-3) which is responsible for the beneficial effect of the Cretan diet (de Lorgeril *et al.*, 1994) is found in greater amounts in the milk of small ruminants, sheep and goats, than in that of bovines.

Cancers

Epidemiology

The absence of hard cheeses in the Mediterranean diet could explain the lower incidence of cancers, since milk, butter and mature cheeses largely contribute to the saturated fat intake. Therefore, it can be conceived that certain studies describe these foods as a risk factor, each time that cancers are associated with energy consumption or obesity such as cancer of the colon or hormone-dependent cancers (Richardson et al., 1991; reviewed in Clavel-Chapelon et al., 1996; Gerber, 1996c; Gerber et al., 1996b). However, this has also been recently described for lung cancer (de Stefani et al., 1997).

On the other hand, it seems that fermented milk reduces the risk of breast cancer (Lé et al., 1986; Van't Veer et al., 1989). The most recent study showed a protection against breast cancer by milk products, without differentiating the origin (Knekt et al., 1996). Two case-control studies also showed a protection effect by fermented milk for cancer of the colon (Adersson-Hassam and Astier-Dumas, 1991; Boutron et al., 1996), this effect was not found in a prospective Dutch study (Kampman et al., 1994).

Mechanisms

Soft cheeses provide fewer lipids and in particular saturated fatty acids than hard cheeses (therefore the risk of developing the insulin-resistant syndrome is lower).

Fermented milk might be a protector against breast cancer, by inducing a colon flora that favours faecal excretion of oestrogens and eventually the conversion of phyto-oestrogen precursors into phyto-oestrogens.

Osteoporosis

Given the moderate calcium intake (not more than 800 mg per day), the Mediterranean diet could increase the risk of osteoporosis in menopausal women. Calcium is the principal component of bone, and it is essential that the intake be greater than the loss, especially during growth, pregnancy and lactation. However, opinions diverge with respect to the need for large supplementary calcium intake (reviewed in Corpet and Gerber, 1996). This could explain why a large ingestion of milk in adults does not significantly reduce the incidence of fractures. Indeed, the incidence of fractures is low in populations that ingest fairly little calcium (Japan, Mediterranean countries). The entire set of epidemiological results do not demonstrate that the consumption of dairy products protects against fractures. However, generally in rich societies, the consumption of milk products is associated to a sedentary life style, as well as a major consumption of animal protein: therefore it is very difficult to exclude these confusion factors.

In Mediterranean countries, the incidence of hip fractures was clearly lower than in Northern European countries in the 1960-1970s (20 to 50 cases versus 100 to 200 cases per year for 100,000). However, recently an increase in the number of fractures is observed, concomitant with an increase in the consumption of milk products. Greece has seen the incidence of hip fractures in menopausal women increase by 50% between 1960 and 1990, while the availability of dairy products commercialised doubled.

However, when calcium is combined with vitamin D, there is a reduction in fractures due to osteoporosis in the elderly (Chapuy *et al.*, 1992). Therefore, it is possible that the Mediterranean sunshine levels is as important in the reduction of fracture incidence as the low calcium and protein intake. Indeed, the comparison of the levels of fractures due to osteoporosis was performed between countries with a low calcium and protein consumption and a sunny climate (Mediterranean countries), and countries with a high calcium and protein consumption, with little sun (Great Britain and Norway) (Abelow *et al.*, 1992).

Olive oil

Cardiovascular diseases

Fatty acids
Generally the low risk of coronary heart disease in Mediterranean countries has been associated with the consumption of olive oil (Keys *et al.*, 1986).

> However, in diet manipulation studies (Mensink *et al.*, 1992) the other poly-unsaturated fatty acid rich vegetable oils (sunflower, corn) induce a greater decrease in the level of LDL-cholesterol than olive oil, mainly composed of oleic acid, a mono-unsaturated fatty acid. On the other hand, the level of HDL-cholesterol is unchanged or even increased with the latter, contrary to the former (Yu *et al.*, 1995), which makes this type of intervention preferable. It has been demonstrated that the levels of oleic acid in cholesterol esters was associated to HDL cholesterol levels (Sandker, 1993). It would seem that oleic acid is neutral with respect to LDL-cholesterol but preserves HDL cholesterol, which is beneficial in the context of low cholesterol intake. However, a high cholesterol intake accompanies mono-unsaturated fatty acids of animal origin (40% in beef and 45% in pork; Gerber, 1995) and in this case, the diet must include a certain proportion of poly-unsaturated fatty acids to maintain cholesterolemia at a satisfactory level (Hayes *et al.*, 1992). This situation is found in the South West of France where a high mono-unsaturated fatty acid intake (goose and duck fat, pork meat) is accompanied by the frequent use of sunflower oil (Gerber *et al.*, 1998).

Is the Mediterranean diet with its predominant olive oil intake sufficient to cover the essential fatty acid (linoleic acid for the n-6 series and α-linolenic for the n-3 series) intake given the use of mainly olive oil? Even though it is relatively low in poly-unsaturated fatty acids, if olive oil is 25% of the lipid intake, its contribution in linoleic acid is sufficient to reach the recommended allowance for this essential fatty acid, *i.e.* 2 to 3% of calorie intake (Kushi *et al.*, 1995 and chapter "Olive oil, olive oil by-products and olive fruit"). The low α-linolenic intake (< 1%) of olive oil is compensated by the vegetable and meat intake from animals fed on these vegetables.

Other components
As vegetable oils are mainly composed of unsaturated fatty acids, they often contain natural anti-oxidants. Thus sunflower oil is very rich in vitamin E (60 mg/100 g). Olive oil only contains 10 to 12 mg/100 g of vitamin E but it has other anti-oxidants: phenolic compounds (oleuropein and hydroxytyrosol). It has been shown (Visioli and Galli, 1998) that hydroxy-

tyrosol protected the consumption of vitamin E in LDLs undergoing oxidative stress *in vitro*, and decreased the formation of conjugated dienes (*also see the chapter* "Olive oil, olive oil by-products and olive fruit").

Finally, it should be noted that even though it is not strictly speaking oil, almonds that are a traditional component of Mediterranean diet, especially in pastries and confectionery, associated with honey, are very rich in mono-unsaturated fatty acids and in fibres, and that this is an optimal combination for the reduction of LDL-cholesterol levels (Abbey *et al.*, 1994).

Cancers

Epidemiology

Recent studies (Martin-Moreno *et al.*, 1994; Trichopoulou *et al.*, 1995) showed that a large olive oil intake reduced the risk of breast cancer. The Italian study cited above (Franceschi *et al.*, 1996; Favero *et al.*, 1998) showed a modest effect of olive oil, smaller than that of other vegetable oils, while in the same countries another team found an inverse association with lung cancer (Fortes *et al.*, 1995). A case-control study on cancer of the colon carried out in Mediterranean countries (Benito *et al.*, 1990) did not show any association with fat intake (mainly olive oil).

Mechanisms

Contrary to cardiovascular diseases, it is not clear whether that mono-unsaturated fatty acids are involved in the protective effect for breast cancer. Mono-unsaturated fatty acids are a risk factor in studies where the lipid intake increases the estimated relative risk (reviewed by Gerber and Richardson, 1995). The latter do not seem significantly protective in these studies or in prospective studies except in the first analysis of the Nurses' Health Study (Willet *et al.*, 1992) and recently in the study by Wolk *et al.*, (1992). However in the latter study, the protective effect of mono-unsaturated fatty acids is only significant after application of special statistical models (mutual adjustment over the different fatty acid classes, calculation of continuous OR).

It has been seen that olive oil also contains phenolic compounds that are also present in many plant products, and have been described as protectors. It is possible that these compounds are also responsible for the beneficial effect of olive oil on cancers.

Finally, the fact that olive oil may appear as protective against certain cancers cannot be disregarded, since it is inversely correlated with the use of saturated fats, butter and cream. A study has shown that the ingestion of olive oil instead of butter decreases the insulin peak (Rasmussen *et al.*, 1996), which could decrease the risk of seeing insulin-resistance appear with its ensuing hormone alterations, which are risk factors for hormone-dependent cancers (*see above*).

Wine

Cardiovascular diseases

Epidemiology

There is an increasing amount of evidence suggesting that a moderate alcohol consumption is associated with a decrease in the risk of infarction (reviewed in Corpet and Gerber, 1997). A North American study (Rehm *et al.*, 1997) showed that if the risk of cardiovascular disease does not increase in male heavy drinkers, in women the risk increases from 4 glasses of alcoholic drinks per day. The enormous study (490 000 men and women in the United States) by Thun *et al.* (1997), showed that the protection related to alcoholic drinks is limited to persons older than 60 years presenting a risk of cardiovascular disease and with a consumption not exceeding 4 glasses of alcoholic beverages per day. Some studies tend to show that wine has a superior effect to that of other alcoholic beverages (Stampfer *et al.*, 1988, Gronbaek *et al.*, 1995). However, in these studies the wine consuming population represent special groups for whom it is difficult to control all the possible confusion factors (dietary behaviour, life style, physical activity). Some (Renaud, 1992) have even wanted to see in wine consumption the explanation for the "French paradox", according to which cardiovascular mortality is particularly low in France, in spite of high cholesterolemia and lipid intake. This notion of French paradox is questioned on the basis of the exactitude of mortality certificates (Ducimetierre and Richard, 1992), or the adjustment on confusion factors (Criqui and Ringel, 1994); or even the real consumption in fats at the time of any beginning of cardiovascular risk (Law and Wald, 1999).

Mechanisms

It has been shown that a moderate alcohol intake increased HDL cholesterol while decreasing the transfer of cholesterol esters from HDL particles to LDL particles (Fumeron *et al.*, 1995). Alcohol could have a beneficial effect on coagulation and platelet aggregation factors, and on fibrinogen (Hendricks *et al.*, 1994).

The protective effect most closely related to wine could be due to the anti-oxidant phenolic micro-constituents (see chapter "Consumption of wine and prevention of cardiovascular diseases"). Furthermore, a comparison between beer drinkers and wine drinkers showed that only the former develop an android type obesity, which was seen above to be a risk factor for cardiovascular diseases (Duncan *et al.*, 1995; see also box). It also seems that the threshold value of gamma-glutamyl-transferase (GGT) is higher when the alcohol ingested comes from wine (Hoffmeister *et al.*, 1999; and box GGT and MONICA, following pages).

Gamma-glutamyl-transferase (GGT)

GGT is an enzyme that increases with alcohol consumption and is a risk marker for alcohol related pathologies. This increase is linear up to a threshold, from which an exponential increase is observed: this threshold was determined to be 26.3 g/day for alcohol from non specific origin, 41.6 when it is alcohol provided by the consumption of beer and at 50.8 when it is alcohol provided by the consumption of wine (Hoffmeister *et al.*, 1999).

The habit of drinking wine with meals may also be one of the explanation of the possible superiority of wine over alcohol, with respect to cardiovascular diseases. The traditional consumption of wine in Mediterranean countries of Southern France is remarkable by the consistency between subjects both for the quantity and the regular consumption (Gerber *et al.* 1998).

To advise the general public to consume wine even moderately, remains a difficult exercise because the limit that depends on numerous parameters (sex, weight, genetic polymorphism of the enzymatic system) is difficult to fix, and because alcohol induces social risks (road accidents and other types of violence) and other pathologies, including some cancers *(see below)*.

Results of MONICA-France

Pierre Ducimetierre recently reported results concerning the populations of Lille, Strasbourg and Toulouse, characterised by highly varied "wine" or "non wine" alcohol consumption. They indicate that below a daily intake of 40 g of alcohol, plasma parameters such as triglyceridemia, the level of gamma-glutamyl-trasnferase (GGT) indicator of hepatic disorder, blood pressure and the height/hip ratio (H/H, the best currently known anthropometrical indicator of CV risk) are not modified while the HDL cholesterol (HDL-C) increases from the lowest alcohol intake. The examination compared the effects of "wine" alcohol and "non wine" alcohol to doses ≤ 40g/day did not show any difference with respect to HDL-C (thus confirming once again that the HDL-C increase is really due to alcohol), and on the other hand showed a significant increase of GGT and H/H ratio only with "non wine" alcohol.

Cancers

In the cases of cancers, alcohol in any alcoholic beverage form is a **convincing** risk factor, which appears from 120 g/day and increases significantly with dose for epithelial cancers of the upper digestive tract, and also of the pancreas, but less coherently (reviewed in Silverman, 1995; Launoy *et al.*, 1997). These diseases have a higher incidence in regions where hard liquor is consumed. However, a recent study in Denmark (Gronbaek *et al.*, 1998) seems to indicate that only the consumption of beer and hard liquor increases the risk of upper aero-digestive tract. However, there was no adjustment of the risk by food intake. In two Mediterranean countries, Northern Italy (Talamini *et al.*) and Southern France (Richardson *et al.*, 1989), which have a comparable consumption mode, wine was identified as a breast cancer risk factor, like alcohol in other countries, for a consumption of 7 glasses/day. This risk, which increases with dose, is therefore considered as **probable** for breast cancer.

Thus, while wine consumption and risk of cardiovascular disease are associated according to a U or J dose-effect relationship, implicating a beneficial effect for a moderate dose, for cancers the relationship is a straight line that shows that the risk increases linearly with the dose.

Conclusion

This entire review shows that the Mediterranean diet probably constitutes a balanced dietary pattern which is very favourable to individual health. However, spatial and temporal limits of the observations reported must be emphasised.

Spatial limit

Mediterranean countries benefit from a sunny climate, and the health benefits of outdoor life and exposure of the skin to the sun, for individuals who have an adequate melanin synthesis are probable. Thus, regular sun exposure, which favours the synthesis of active vitamin D in the skin induces a possible protection against osteoporosis and some cancers.

Benefits and risks of sun exposure

Mediterraneans with dark skin and hair, denoting melanin synthesis that protects against the carcinogenic effect of UV, can profit from the sun with a lower risk in order to increase vitamin D synthesis, whose beneficial effect in calcium fixation by bone tissue is known, and its anti-carcinogenic effect is strongly suspected. On the contrary, certain Nordic origin populations with blue eyes, or even more, red hair, synthesise little melanin or a bad quality melanin and will be subjected to the carcinogenic effect of UVs by exposing themselves to the sun.

Temporal limit

In most cases, the effects observed correspond to the traditional version of Mediterranean diet, the diet of a society, now partly gone, where time was found to grow and cook a large variety of vegetables and herbs. It is found in rural and poor countries. It can be thought that the health benefits come partly from a restricted caloric intake, and sustained physical expenditure. Elderly rural Mediterraneans are small in comparison with young people from any country, or with the elderly from the Northern countries. Limited energy intake, and considerable physical effort before the end of growth, partly explain this limited size. Physical activity that increases energy expenditure and opposes itself to excess weight, may play a role in low incidence of cardiovascular disease and cancer, together with the Mediterranean type of diet.

This traditional version has largely disappeared, and with it the favourable figures in certain health indicators: cholesterol level, incidence of certain cancers, incidence of fractures. The challenge of prevention by dietary recommendations is therefore double: maintain good habits in Mediterranean countries and export the model to the rest of the occidental countries.

Nothing can be done about the amount of sun in a country, but can cultural habits be influenced, and to what extent?

The results of a survey carried out in the Herault, MEDHEA showed first that dietary traditions vary from one Mediterranean region to another. In the elderly population in the rural Herault, all the Mediterranean diet characteristics are found. However, in the young, and in urban population the results showed that the model tends to disappear. Therefore, the socio-economic context appears as a major determinant: the diet in urban and suburban Montpellier, highly urban, is different from that of other more isolated areas of the department (Gerber *et al.*, 1998; Scali *et al.*, 2000).

Therefore, it is conceivable that in order to extend the Mediterranean model, which might be of paramount importance in Public Health, socio-economic considerations must be associated with nutrition, health and prevention objectives: the challenge is to adapt to modern life conditions a culinary culture which traditionally required a large variety of fresh products and lots of time to cook them.

REFERENCES

- Abbey M, Nestel PJ, Baghurst PA. Antioxidant vitamins and low-density-lipoprotein oxidation. *Am J Clin Nutr* 1993 ; 58 : 525-32.

- Abbey M, Noakes M, Belling B, Nestel PJ. Partial replacement of saturated fatty acids with almonds or walnutslowers plasma cholesterol and low density lipoprotein cholesterol. *Am J Clin Nutr* 1994 ; 59 : 995-9.

- Abelow BJ, *et al.* Cross-cultural association between dietary animal protein and hip fracture : a hypothesis. *Calcif Tissue Int* 1992 ; 50 : 14-8.

- Adler AJ, Holub BJ. Effect of garlic and fish-oil supplementation on serum lipid and lipoprotein concentrations in hypercholesterolemic men. *Am J Clin Nutr* 1997 ; 65 : 445-50.

- Adlercreutz H, Honjo H, Higashi A, *et al.* Urinary excretion of lignans and isoflavonoid phytoestrogens in Japanese men and women consuming a traditional Japanese diet. *Am J Clin Nutr* 1991 ; 54 : 1093-100.

- Agudo A, Esteve MG, Pallares C, Martinez-Ballarin I, Fabregat X, Malats N, MacHengs I, Badia A, Gonzalez CA. Vegetable and fruit intake and the risk of lung cancer in women in Barcelona, Spain. *Eur J Cancer* 1997 ; 33 : 1256-61.

- Alberts DS, Ritenbaugh C, Story JA, Aickin M, Rees-McGee S, Buller MK, Atwood J, Phelps J, Ramanujam PS, Bellapravalu S, Patel J, Bettinger L, Clark L. Randomized, double-blinded, placebo-controlled study of effect of wheat bran fiber and calcium on fecal bile acids in patients with resected adenomatous colon polyps. *J Natl Cancer Inst* 1996 ; 88 : 81-92.

- Ambrosone CB, Kadlubar FF. Toward an integrated approach to molecular epidemiology. *Am J Epidemiol* 1997 ; 146 : 912-8.

- Andersson-Hassam E, Astier-Dumas M. Habitudes alimentaires et cancers colorectaux : étude cas-témoins. *Med Nutr* 1991 ; 27 : 300-4.

- Artaud-Wild SM, Connor WE, Secton G. Differences in coronary mortality can be explain by differences in cholesterol and saturated fat intakes in 40 countries but not in France and Finland. A paradox. *Circulation* 1993 ; 88 : 2771-9.

- Ascherio A, Willet WC, Rimm EB, Giovannucci EL, Stampfer MJ. Dietary iron intake and risk of coronary heart disease among men. *Circulation* 1994 ; 89 : 974-6.

- Baghurst PA, Rohan TH. Dietary fiber and risk of benign proliferative epithelial disorders of the breast. *Int J Cancer* 1995 ; 63 : 481-5.

- Barnard RJ, Ugianskis EJ, Martin DA, Inkeles SB. Role of diet and exercise in the management of hyperinsulinemia and associated atherosclerotic risk factors. *Am J Cardiol* 1992 ; 69 : 440-4.

- Benito E, Obrador A, Stiggelbout A, *et al.* A population-based case-control study of colo-rectal cancer in Majorca. I-Dietray factors. *Int J Cancer* 1990 ; 45 : 69-76.

- Biesalski HK, Bueno de Mesquita B, Chesson A, Chytil F, Grinble R, Hermus RIJ, Kohrle J, Lotan R, Norpoth K, Pastorino U, Thurnham D. Consensus statement on lung cancer. *Eur J Cancer Prev* 1997 ; 6 : 316-22.

- Bingham SA, Atkinson C, Liggins J, Bluck L, Coward A. Phyto-oestrogens : where are we now ? *Br J Nutr* 1998 ; 79 : 393-406.

- Blache D, Gesquière L, Loreau N, Durand P. Oxidant stress : the role of nutrients in cell-lipoprotein interactions. *Proc Nutrition Soc* 1999 ; 58 : 559-63.

- Blot WJ, Li JY, Taylor Ph R, Guo W, *et al*. Nutrition intervention trials in Linxian, China : supplementation with specific vitamin/mineral combinations, cancer incidence, and disease-specific mortality in the general population. *J Natl Cancer Inst* 1993 ; 85 : 1483-92.

- Bohlke K, Spiegelman D, Trichopoulou A, Katsouyanni K, Trichopoulos D. Vitamins A, C and E and the risk of breast cancer : results from a case-control study in Greece. *Br J Cancer* 1999 ; 79 : 23-9.

- Bougnoux P, Corpet D, Gerber M. *Acides gras alimentaires et cancerogenèse. Alimentation et cancer*. Paris : Tec Doc, Lavoisier, 1996 : 281-314.

- Boutron MC, Faivre J, Marteau P, Couillault C, Senesse P, Quipourt V. Calcium, phosphorus, vitamin D, dairy products and colorectal carcinogenesis : a French case-control study. *Br J Cancer* 1996 ; 74 : 145-51.

- Carbonneau MA, Leger CL, Monnier L, Bonnet C, Michel F, Fouret G, Dedieu F, Descomps B. Supplementation with red wine phenolics increases the antioxidant capacity of plasma and vitamin E of low density lipoprotein without changing the lipoprotein Cu2+-oxidability : possible explanation by phenolics location. *Eur J Clin Nutr* 1997 ; 51 : 682-90.

- Carpenter KL, Cheeseman KH, Van Der Veen C, Taylor SE, Walker MK, Mitchinson MJ. Depletion of alpha-tocopherol in human atherosclerotic lesions. *Free Radic Res* 1995 ; 23 : 549-58.

- Cassidy A, Bingham S, Setchell KDR. Biological effects of a diet of soy protein rich in isoflavones on the menstrual cycle of premenopausal women. *Am J Clin Nutr* 1994 ; 60 : 333-40.

- Chapuy MC, *et al*. Vitamin D3 and calcium to prevent hip fractures in elderly women. *N Engl J Med* 1992 ; 327 : 1637-42.

- Clavel-Chapelon F, Niravong M, Joseph RR. Diet and breast cancer : review of the epidemiologic literature. *Cancer Detect Prev* 1997 ; 21 : 426-40.

- Clavel-Chapelon F, Van Liere M, Dormoy N. Cancer du sein et alimentation. *Alimentation et cancers. Evaluation scientifique*. In : Riboli E, Decloitre F, Collet-Ribbing C, eds. Paris : Tec Doc, Lavoisier, 1996 : 157-202.

- Comstock GW, Alberg AJ, Huang HY, Wu K, Burke AE, Hoffman SC, Norkus EP, Gross M, Cutler RG, Morris JS, Spate VL, Helzlsouer KJ. The risk of developing lung cancer associated with antioxidants in the blood : ascorbic acid, carotenoids, alpha-tocopherol, selenium, and total peroxyl radical absorbing capacity. *Cancer Epidemiol Biomark Prev* 1997 ; 6 : 907-16.

- Corpet DE, Gerber M. Alimentation méditerranéenne et santé. I. Caractéristiques. Maladies cardiovasculaires et autres affections. *Med Nutr* 1997 ; 4 : 129-42.

- Corti MC, Gaziano M, Hennekens CH. Review : iron status and risk of cardiovascular disease. *Ann Epidemiol* 1997 ; 7 : 62-8.

- Criqui MH, Ringel BL. Does diet or alcohol explain the french paradox ? *Lancet* 1994 ; 344 : 1719-23.

- D'Avanzo B, Ron E, La Vecchia C, Franceschi S, Negri E. Selected micronutrient intake and thyroid carcinoma risk. *Cancer* 1997 ; 79 : 2186-92.

- Daviglus ML, Stamler J, Orencia AJ, Dyer AR, Liu K, Greenland P, Walsh MK, Morris D, Shekelle RB. Fish consumption and the 30-year risk of fatal myocardial infarction. *N Engl J Med* 1997 ; 336 : 1046-53.

- De Klerk NH, Musk AW, Ambrosini GL, Eccles JL, Hansen J, Olsen N, Watts VL, Lund HG, Pang SC, Beilby J, Hobbs MS. Vitamin A and cancer prevention II : comparison of the effects of retinol and beta-carotene. *Int J Cancer* 1998 ; 75 : 362-7.

- De Lorgeril M, Renaud S, Mamelle N, *et al*. Mediterranean alpha-linolenic acid rich diet in secondary pevention of coronary heart disease. *Lancet* 1994 ; 343 : 1454-9.

- De Stefani E, Correa P, Ronco A, Mendilaharsu M, Guidobono M, Deneo-Pellegrini H. Die-

• tary fiber and risk of breast cancer: a case-control study in Uruguay. *Nutr Cancer* 1997; 28: 14-9.

• De Stefani E, Fontham ETH, Chen V, *et al.* Fatty foods and the risk of lung cancer: a case-control study from Uruguay. *Int J Cancer* 1997; 71: 760-6.

• De Cosse J, Miller HH, Lesser ML. Effect of wheat fiber and vitamins C and E on rectal polyps in patients with familial adenomatous polyposis. *J Natl Cancer Inst* 1993; 81: 1290-7.

• Diaz MN, Frei B, Vita JA, Keaney JF. Antioxidants and atherosclerotic heart disease. *N Engl J Med* 1997; 337: 408-16.

• Dorgan JF, Sowell A, Swanson CA, Potischman N, Miller R, Scussler N, Stephenson HE. Relationships of serum carotenoids, retinol, alpha-tocopherol, and selenium with breast cancer risk: results from a prospective study in Columbia, Missouri. *Cancer Causes Control* 1998; 9: 89-97.

• Ducimetierre P, Richard JL. Dietary lipids and coronary heart disease: is there a French paradox. *Nutr Metab Cardiovasc Dis* 1992; 2: 195-201.

• Duncan BB, Chambless LE, Schmidt MI, Folsom AR, Szklo M, Crouse JR, Carpenter MA. Association of the waist-to-hip ratio is different with wine than with beer or hard liquor consumption. Atherosclerosis risk in community study investigators. *Am J Epidemiol* 1995; 142: 1034-8.

• Eichholzer M, Stahelin HB, Gey KF, Ludin E, Bernasconi F. Prediction of male cancer mortality by plasma levels of interacting vitamins: 17-year follow-up of the prospective Basel study. *Int J Cancer* 1996; 66: 145-50.

• ECP Consensus panel on cereals and cancer: consensus meeting on cereals, fibre and colorectal and breast cancers. *Eur J Cancer Prev* 1997b; 6: 512-4.

• Favero A, Parpinel M, Franceschi S. Diet and risk of breast cancer: major findings from an Italian case-control study. *Biomed Pharmacother* 1998; 52: 109-15.

• Fontham ETH. Vitamin-C, vitamin-C rich foods, and cancer-epidemiologic studies. In: Frei B, ed. *Natural antioxidants in human health and disease.* New York: Academic Press, 1994.

• Fortes C, Forastiere F, Anatra F, Schmid G. Consumption of olive oil and specific food groups in relation to breast cancer risk in Greece. *J Natl Cancer Inst* 1995; 87: 1020-1.

• Fotsis T, Pepper MS, Aktas E, Breit S, Rasku S, Adlercreutz H, Wahala K, Montesano R, Schweigerer L. Flavonoids, dietary-derived inhibitors of cell proliferation and *in vitro* angiogenesis. *Cancer Res* 1997; 57: 2916-21.

• Franceschi S, Bidoli E, La Vecchia C, Talamini E, d'Avanzo B, Negri E. Tomatoes and risk of digestive tracts cancers. *Int J Cancer* 1994; 59: 181-4.

• Franceschi S, Favero A, La Vecchia C, *et al.* Influence of food groups and food diversity on breast cancer in Italy. *Int J Cancer* 1995; 63: 785-9.

• Franceschi S, Favero A, Decarli A, La Vecchia C, Ferraroni M, Russo A, Salvini S, Amadori D, Conti E, Montella M, Giacosa A. Intake of macronutrients and risk of breast cancer. *Lancet* 1996; 347: 1351-6.

• Franceschi S, Parpinel M, La Vecchia C, Favero A, Talamini R, Negri E. Role of different types of vegetables and fruit in the prevention of cancer of the colon, rectum, and breast. *Epidemiology* 1998-a; 9: 338-41.

• Franceschi S, Favero A, Parpinel M, Giacosa A, La Vecchia C. Italian study on colorectal cancer with emphasis on influence of cereals. *Eur J Cancer Prev* 1998b; 7S: S19-S23.

• Franceschi S, La Vecchia C, Russo A, Favero A, Negri E, Conti E, Montella M, Filiberti R, Amadori D, Decarli A. Macronutrient intake and risk of colorectal cancer in Italy. *Int J Cancer* 1998c; 76: 321-4.

• Franceschi S, Favero A, Conti E, Talamini R, Volpe R, Negri E, Barzan L, La Vecchia C. Food groups, oils and butter, and cancer of the oral cavity and pharynx. *Br J Cancer* 1999; 80(3/4): 614-20.

• Freudenheim JL, Marsall JR, Vena JE, Laughlin R, Brasure J, Swanson MK, Nemoto T, Graham S. Premenopausal breast cancer risk and intake of vegetables, fruits, and related nutrients. *J Natl Cancer Inst* 1996; 88: 340-8.

• Fumeron F, Betoulle D, Gerald L, *et al.* Alcohol intake modulates the effect of a polymorphism of the choleseryl ester transfer protein gene on plasma high density lipoprotein and the risk of myocardial infarction. *J Clin Invest* 1995 ; 96 : 1664-71.

• Galanis DJ, Kolonel LN, Lee J, Nomura A. Intakes of selected foods and beverages and the incidence of gastric cancer among the Japanese residents of Hawaii : a prospective study. *Int J Epidemiol* 1998 ; 27 : 173-80.

• Gann PH, Hennekens CH, Sacks FM, Grodstein F, Giovannucci E, Stampfer MJ. Prospective study of plasma fatty acids and risk of prostate cancer. *J Natl Cancer Inst* 1994 ; 86 : 281-6.

• Gann PH, Ma J, Giovannucci E, Willett W, Sacks FM, Hennekens CH, Stampfer MJ. Lower prostate cancer risk in men with elevated plasma lycopene levels : results of a prospective analysis. *Cancer Res* 1999 ; 59 : 1225-30.

• Garcia-Closas R, Gonzalez CA, Agudo A, Riboli E. Intake of specific carotenoids and flavonoids and the risk of gastric cancer in Spain. *Cancer Causes Control* 1999 ; 10 : 71-5.

• Gates JR, Parpia B, Campbell TC, Junshi C. Association of dietary factors and selected plasma variables with sex-hormone-binding globulin in rural Chinese women. *Am J Clin Nutr* 1996 ; 63 : 22-31.

• Gaziano JM, Manson JE, Branch LG, *et al*. A prospective study of consumption of carotenoids in fruits and vegetables and decreased cardiovascular mortality in the elderly. *Ann Epidemiol* 1995 ; 5 : 255-60.

• Gerber M. Fat in the mediterranean diet. *Int J Nutr Vit Res* 1995 ; 65 : 59-60.

• Gerber M. Fiber and breast cancer : another piece of the puzzle – but still an incomplete picture. *J Natl Cancer Inst* 1996 a ; 88 : 857-8.

• Gerber M. Vitamine E, selenium et cancers. In : Decloitre F, Riboli E, Collet-Ribbing C, eds. *Alimentation et Cancers. Évaluation scientifique*. Paris : Tec-Doc, Lavoisier, 1996b : 345-72.

• Gerber M. Alimentation et cancer de l'endomètre. In : Decloitre F, Riboli E, Collet-Ribbing C, eds. *Alimentation et Cancers. Évaluation scientifique*. Paris : Tec-Doc, Lavoisier, 1996c : 213-22.

• Gerber M. Fibre and breast cancer. *Eur J Cancer Prev* 1998 ; 7S : S63-S67.

• Gerber M, Astre C, Segala C, Saintot M, Scali J, Simony-Lafontaine J, Grenier J, Pujol H. Oxidant-antioxidant status alterations in cancer patients : relationship to tumor progression. *J Nutr* 1996 a ; 126 : 1201S-7S.

• Gerber M, Astre C, Ségala C, Saintot M, Scali J, Simony-Lafontaine J, Grenier J, Pujol H. Tumor progression and oxidant-anti-oxidant status. *Cancer Lett* 1997 ; 114 : 211-4.

• Gerber M, Bougnoux P, Corpet D. Équilibre énergétique et cancers. In : Decloitre F, Riboli E, Collet-Ribbing C, eds. *Alimentation et Cancers. Évaluation scientifique*. Paris : Tec-Doc, Lavoisier, 1996 b : 255-80.

• Gerber M, Corpet D. Alimentation méditerranéenne et Santé. II-Cancers. *Med Nutr* 1997 ; 4 : 143-54.

• Gerber M, Richardson S. Re : consumption of olive oil and specific food groups in relation to breast cancer risk in Greece. *J Natl Cancer Inst* 1995 ; 87 : 1020-2.

• Gerber M, Scali J, Michaud A, Siari S, Grosclaude P, Faliu B. Consommation alimentaire dans le département de l'Hérault, du Tarn, et la zone urbaine de Toulouse. Rapport du Conseil régional LR, 1998 b.

• Gerhardsson-de-Verdier MG, *et al*. Meat, cooking methods and colorectal cancer – a case referent study in Stockholm. *Int J Cancer* 1991 ; 49 : 520-5.

• Gey KF, Puska P. Inverse correlation between plasma vitamin E and mortality from ischemic heart disease in cross-cultural epidemiology. *Am J Clin Nutr* 1991 ; 53 : 326S-34S.

• Ghadirian P, Lacroix A, Maisonneuve P, Perret C, Potvin C, Gravel D, Bernard D, Boyle P. Nutritional factors and colon carcinoma. *Cancer* 1997 ; 80 : 858-64.

• Giovannucci E, Rimm EB, Colditz GA, Stampfer MJ, Ascherio A, Chute CC, Willett WC. A prospective study of dietay fat and risk of prostate cancer. *J Natl Cancer Inst* 1993 ; 85 : 1571-9.

- Giovannucci E, Rimm EB, Stampfer MJ, Colditz GA, Ascherio A, Willett WC. Intake of fat, meat, and fiber in relation to risk of colon cancer in men. *Cancer Res* 1994 ; 54 : 2390-7.

- Giovannucci E, Ascherio A, Rimm EB, Stampfer MJ, Colditz GA, Willett WC. Intake of carotenoids and retinol in relation to risk of prostate cancer. *J Natl Cancer Inst* 1995 ; 87 : 1767-76.

- Giovannucci E, Goldin B. The role of fat, fatty acids, and total energy intake in the etiology of human colon cancer. *Am J Clin Nutr* 1997 ; 66S : 1564S-71S.

- GISSI-prevenzione investigators. Dietary supplementation with n-3 polyunsaturated fatty acids and vitamin E after myocardial infarction : results of the GISSI-prevenzione trial. *Lancet* 1999 ; 354 : 447-55.

- Goldin BR, Adlercreutz H, Gorbach SL, *et al.* Estrogen excretion patterns and plasma levels in vegetarian and omnivorous women. *N Engl J Med* 1982 ; 307 : 1542-7.

- Goldbohm RA, *et al.* A prospective cohort study on the relation between meat consumption and the risk of colon cancer. *Cancer Res* 1994 ; 54 : 718-23.

- Goodman MT, Wilkens LR, Hankin JH, Lyu LC, Wu AH, Kolonel LN. Association of soy and fiber consumption with the risk of endometrial cancer. *Am J Epidemiol* 1997 ; 146 : 294-306.

- Graham S, Hellmann R, Marshall J, *et al.* Nutritional epidemiology of postmenopausal breast cancer in Western New-York. *Am J Epidemiol* 1991 ; 134 : 552-66.

- Gramenzi A, Gentile A, Fasoli M, *et al.* Association between certain foods and the risk of acute myocardial infarction in women. *Br Med J* 1990 ; 300 : 771-3.

- Greenberg ER, Baron JA, Tosteson TD, *et al.* (the polyp prevention study group). A clinical trial of antioxidant vitamins to prevent colorectal adenoma. *N Engl J Med* 1994 ; 331 : 141-7.

- Grievink L, Jansen SMA, Van'T Veer P, Brunekreef B. Acute effects of ozone on pulmonary function of cyclists receiving antioxidant supplements. *Occup Environ Med* 1998 ; 55 : 13-7.

- Grievink L, Zijlstra AG, Ke X, Brunekreef B. Double-blind intervention trial on modulation of ozone effects on pulmonary function by antioxidant supplements. *Am J Epidemiol* 1999 ; 149(4) : 306-14.

- Gronbaek M, *et al.* Mortality associated with moderate intakes of wine, beer or spirits. *Br Med J* 1995 ; 310 : 1165-9.

- Gronbaek M, Becker U, Johansen D, Tonnesen H, Jensen G, Sorensen TIA. Population based cohort study of the association between alcohol intake and cancer of the upper digestive tract. *Br Med J* 1998 ; 317 : 844-8.

- Hankinson SE, Willett WC, Colditz GA, Hunter DJ, Michaud DS, Deroo B, Rosner B, Speizer FE, Pollak M. Circulating concentrations of insulin-like growth factor-I and risk of breast cancer. *Lancet* 1998 ; 351 : 1393-6.

- Harris WS. N-3 fatty acids and serum lipoproteins : human studies. *Am J Clin Nutr* 1997 ; 65 : 1645S-54S.

- Harvei S, Bjerve K, Tretli S, Jellum E, Robsahm TE, Vatten L. Prediagnostic level of fatty acids in serum phospholipids : gamma-3 and gamma-6 fatty acids and the risk of prostate cancer. *Int J Cancer* 1997 ; 71 : 545-51.

- Hayes KC, Koshla P. Dietary fatty acid thresholds and cholesterolemia. *FASEB J* 1992 ; 6 : 2600-7.

- Heinonen OP, Albanes D, Virtamo J, Taylor PR, Huttunen JK, Hartman AM, Haapakoski J, Malila N, Rautalahti M, Ripatti S, Maenpaa H, Teerenhovi L, Koss L, Virolainen M, Edwards BK. Prostate cancer and supplementation with alpha-tocopherol and beta-carotene : incidence and mortality in a controlled trial. *J Natl Cancer Inst* 1998 ; 90 : 440-6.

- Hertog MGL, Feskens EJM, Hollman PCH, Katan MB, Kromhout D. Dietary antioxidants flavonoïds and the risk of coronary heart disease : the Zutphen elderly study. *Lancet* 1993 ; 342 : 1007-11.

- Hertog MGL, Hollman PCH. Potential health effects of the dietary flavonol quercetin. *Eur J Clin Nutr* 1996 ; 50 : 63-71.

- Hertog MGL, Sweetnam PM, Fehily AM, Elwood PC, Kromhout D. Antioxidant flavonols and ischemic heart disease in a Welsh population of men : the Caerphilly Study. *Am J Clin Nutr* 1997 ; 65 : 1489-94.

• Hoffmeister H, Schelp FP, Mensink GBM, Dietz E, Böhning D. The relationship between alcohol consumption, health indicators and mortality in the German population. *Int J Epidemiol* 1999 ; 28 : 1066-72.

• Hopkins KD. Dietary fibre decreases cardiovascular events. *Lancet* 1996 ; 348 : 1648.

• Horn-Ross PL, Morrow M, Ljung BM. Diet and the risk of salivary gland cancer. *Am J Epidemiol* 1997 ; 146 : 171-6.

• Howe GR, Friedenreich Ch M, Jain M, Miller AB. A cohort study of fat intake and risk of breast cancer. *J Natl Cancer Inst* 1991 ; 83 : 336-40.

• Howe GR, *et al.* Dietary intake of fiber and decreased risk of cancers of the colon and rectum – evidence from the combined analysis of 13 case-control studies. *J Natl Cancer Inst* 1992 ; 84 : 1887-96.

• Hsing AW, McLaughlin JK, Chow WH, Schuman LM, Co Chien HT, Gridley G, Bjelke E, Wacholder S, Blot WJ. Risk factors for colorectal cancer in a prospective study among US white men. *Int J Cancer* 1998 ; 77 : 549-53.

• Hylla S, Gostner A, Dusel G, Anger H, Bartram HP, Christl SU, Kasper H, Scheppach W. Effects of resistant starch on the colon in healthy volunteers : possible implications for cancer prevention. *Am J Clin Nutr* 1998 ; 67 : 136-42.

• IARC. *Carotenoids. Handbookds of cancer prevention.* IARC, Lyon, 1998.

• Ingram D, Sanders K, Kolybaba M, Lopez D. Case-control study of phyto-oestrogens and breast cancer. *Lancet* 1997 ; 350 : 990-4.

• Jacobs DR, Slavin J, Marquart L. Whole grain intake and cancer : a review of the litterature. *Nutr Cancer* 1995 ; 24 : 221-9.

• Ji BT, Chow WHO, Yang G, McLaughlin JK, Zheng W, Shu XO, Jin F, Gao RN, Gao YT, Fraumeni JF. Dietary habits and stomach cancer in Shanghai, China. *Int J Cancer* 1998 ; 76 : 659-64.

• Kaaks R, Tuyns AJ, Haelterman M, Riboli E. Nutrient intake patterns and gastric cancer risk : a case-control study in Belgium. *Int J Cancer* 1998 ; 78 : 415-20.

• Kaiser L, Boyd NF, Kriukov V, Tritchler D. Fish consumption and cancer risk : an ecological study. *Nutr Cancer* 1989 ; 12 : 61-8.

• Kampman E, *et al.* Calcium, vitamin D, dairy foods, and the occurrence colorectal adenomas among men and women in two prospective studies. *Am J Epidemiol* 1994 ; 139 : 16-29.

• Key TJ, Silcocks PB, Davey GK, Appleby PN, Bishop DT. A case-control study of diet and prostate cancer. *Br J Cancer* 1997 ; 76 : 678-87.

• Keys A, Fidanza F, Scardi U, *et al.* Studies on serum cholesterol and other characteristics on clinically healthy men in Italy. *Arch Intern Med* 1954a ; 93 : 328-32.

• Keys A, Lorenzo F, Rodriguez Minon VL, *et al.* Studies on the diet, body fatness and serum cholesterol in Madrid, Spain. *Metabolism* 1954b ; 3 : 195-8.

• Keys A, Taylor HL, Blackburn HW, *et al.* The diet and 15 years death rate in Seven Countries Studies. *Am J Epidemiol* 1986 ; 124 : 903-15.

• Knekt P, Albanes D, Seppänen R, *et al.* Dietary fat and risk of breast cancer. *Am J Clin Nutr* 1990 ; 52 : 903-8.

• Knekt P, Reunanen A, Jarvinen R, *et al.* Antioxidant vitamin intake and coronary mortality in a longitudinal population study. *Am J Epidemiol* 1994 a ; 134 : 1180-9.

• Knekt P, Steineck G, Järvinen R, Hakulinen T, Aromaa A. Intake of fried meat and risk of cancer : a follow-up study in Finland. *Int J Cancer* 1994 b ; 59 : 756-60.

• Knekt P, Jarvinen R, Reunanen A, Maatela J. Flavonoid intake and coronary mortality in Finland : a cohort study. *Br Med J* 1996 a ; 312 : 478-81.

• Knekt P, Jarvinen R, Seppanen R, Pukkala E, Aromaa A. Intake of dairy products and the risk of breast cancer. *Br J Cancer* 1996 b ; 73 : 687-91.

• Knekt P, Jarvinen R, Teppo L, Aromaa A, Seppanen R. Role of various carotenoids in lung cancer prevention. *J Natl Cancer Inst* 1999 ; 91 : 182-3.

- Knekt P, Jarvinen R, Seppanen R, Heliovaara M, Teppo L, Pukkala E, Aromaa A. Dietary flavonoids and the risk of lung cancer and other malignant neoplasms. *Am J Epidemiol* 1997 ; 146 : 223-30.

- Kohlmeier L, Dark JD, Gomez-Garcia E, et al. Lycopene and myocardial infarction risk in the Euramic study. *Am J Epidemiol* 1997 ; 146 : 618-26.

- Kromhout D, Bosschieter EB, Coulander CR. The inverse relationship between fish consumption and 20-year mortality from coronary heart disease. *N Engl J Med* 1985 ; 312 : 1205-9.

- Kushi LH, et al. Dietary fat and premenopausal breast cancer. *J Natl Cancer Inst* 1992 ; 84 : 1092-9.

- Kushi LH, Lenart EB, Willett WC. Health implications of mediterranean diets in light of contemporary knowledge. 1. plant foods and dairy products. 2. Meats, wine, fats, and oils. *Am J Clin Nutr* 1995 ; 61 : S1407-S27.

- Kushi LH, Folsom AR, Prineas RJ, Mink PJ, Wu Y, Bostick RM. Dietary antioxidant vitamins and death from coronary heart disease in postmenopausal women. *N Engl J Med* 1996 ; 334 : 1156-62.

- Kushi LH, Mink PJ, Folsom AR, Anderson KE, Zheng W, Lazovich D, Sellers TA. Prospective study of diet and ovarian cancer. *Am J Epidemiol* 1999 ; 149(1) : 21-31.

- La Vecchia C, Braga C, Negri E, Franceschi S, Russo A, Conti E, Falcini F, Giacosa A, Montella M, Decarli A. Intake of selected micronutrients and risk of colorectal cancer. *Int J Cancer* 1997 ; 73 : 525-30.

- La Vecchia C, Chatenoud L. Fibres, whole-grain foods and breast and other cancers. *Eur J Cancer Prev* 1998 ; 7S : S25-S28.

- La Vecchia C, Ferraroni M, Negri E, Franceschi S. Role of various carotenoids in the risk of breast cancer. *Int J Cancer* 1998 ; 75 : 482-3.

- Landmark K, Abdelnoor M, Kilhovd B, Dorum HP. Eating fish may reduce infarct size and the occurrence of Q wave infarcts. *Eur J Clin Nutr* 1998 ; 52 : 40-4.

- Launoy G, Milan C, Day NE, Faivre J, Pienkowski P, Gignoux M. Oesophageal cancer in France : potential importance of hot alcoholic drinks. *Int J Cancer* 1997 ; 71 : 917-23.

- Le Marchand, et al. Animal fat consumption and prostate cancer : a prospective study in Hawaii. *Epidemiology* 1994 ; 5 : 276-82.

- Lé MG, Moulton LH, Hill C, Kramar A. Consumption of dairy produce and alcohol in a case-control study of breast cancer. *J Natl Cancer Inst* 1986 ; 77 : 633-6.

- Lee HP, Gourley L, Duffy SW, et al. Dietary effects on breast-cancer risk in Singapore. *Lancet* 1991 ; 337 : 1197-200.

- Levi F, La Vecchia C, Gulie C, Negri E. Dietary factors and breast cancer risk in Vaud, Switzerland. *Nutr Cancer* 1993 ; 19 : 327-35.

- Levi F, Pasche C, La Vecchia C, Lucchini F, Franceschi S. Food groups and colorectal cancer risk. *Br J Cancer* 1999 ; 79 : 1283-7.

- Lewis SJ, Heaton KW, Oakey RE, McGarrigle HHG. Lower serum oestrogen concentrations associated with faster intestinal transit. *Br J Cancer* 1997 ; 76 : 395-400.

- Lihavainen L, Korpela R. Conjugated linoleic acid. Scand. *J Nutr* 1998 ; 42 : 74-6.

- Linn S, Caroll M, Johnson C, Fulwood R, Kalsbeecek W, Briefel R. HDL-Cholesterol and alcohol consumption in US white end Black adults : data from NHANES II. *Am J Public Health* 1993 ; 83 : 811-6.

- Liu, Stampfer MJ, Hu FB, Giovannucci E, Rimm E, Manson JE, Hennekens CH, Willet WC. Whole-grain consumption and risk of coronary heart disease : results from the Nurses'Health Study. *Am J Clin Nutr* 1999 ; 70 : 412-9.

- London S, Willett WC, Longcope C, McKinlay S. Alcohol and other dietary factors in relation to serum hormone concentrations in women at climateric. *Am J Clin Nutr* 1991 ; 53 : 166-71.

- Longnecker MP, Nexcomb PA, Mittendorf R, Greenberg R, Willett WC. Intake of carrots, spinach, and supplements containing vitamin A in relation to risk of breast cancer. *Cancer Epidemiol Biom Prev* 1997 ; 6 : 887-92.

- Mac Lennan R, Macrae F, Bian C, et al. Randomized trial of intake of fat, fiber, and beta-carotene to prevent colorectal adenomas. *J Natl Cancer Inst* 1995 ; 87 : 1760-6

• Mantzoros CS, Tzonou A, Signorello LB, Stampfer M, Trichopoulos D, Adami HO. Insulin-like growth factor 1 in relation to prostate cancer and benign prostatic hyperplasia. *Br J Cancer* 1997 ; 76 : 1115-8.

• Marckmann P, Gronbaek M. Fish consumption and coronary heart disease mortality. A systematic review of prospective cohort studies. *Eur J Clin Nutr* 1999 ; 53 : 585-90.

• Martin-Moreno JM, Willet WC, Gorgojo L, *et al*. Dietary fat, olive oil intake and breast cancer risk. *Int J Cancer* 1994 ; 58 : 774-80.

• McKeon-Eyssen G, Holloway C, Jazmaji V, Bright-See E, Dion P, Bruce WR. A randomized trial of vitamins C and E in the prevention of recurrence of colorectaal polyps. *Cancer Res* 1988 ; 48 : 4701-5.

• McKeon-Essen G, *et al*. A randomized trial of a low fat high fibre diet in the recurrence of colorectal polyps. *J Clin Epidemiol* 1994 ; 47 : 525-36.

• Meflah K, Cherbut C, Riboli E, Kaaks R, Corpet D. Fibres alimentaires et cancer colorectal. In : Riboli E, Decloitre F *et al.*, eds. *Alimentation et cancer*. Paris : Tec Doc, Lavoisier, 1996 ; 402-25.

• Mensink RP, Katan MB. Effect of dietary fatty acids on serum lipids and lipoproteins. A meta-analysis of 27 trials. *Arterioscler Thromb* 1992 ; 12 : 911-9.

• Mezzetti M, La Vecchia C, Decarli A, Boyle P, Talamini R, Franceschi S. Population attributable risk for breast cancer : diet, nutrition, and physical exercise. *J Natl Cancer Inst* 1998 ; 90 : 389-94.

• Michaud DS, Spiegelman D, Clinton SK, Rimm EB, Willett WC, Giovannucci EL. Fruit and vegetable intake and incidence of bladder cancer in a male prospective cohort. *J Natl Cancer Inst* 1999 ; 91(7) : 605-13.

• Micozzi MS, Brown ED, Edwards BK, *et al*. Plasma carotenoïd response to chronic intake of selected foods and beta-carotene supplements in mes. *Am J Clin Nutr* 1992 ; 55 : 1120-5.

• Mills PK, *et al*. Cohort study of diet lifestyle and prostate cancer in Adventist men. *Cancer* 1989 ; 64 : 598-604.

• Mori TA, Vandongen R, Beilin LJ, *et al*. Effects of varying fat, fish and fishoils on blood lipids in a randomized controlled trial in me at risk of heart disease. *Am J Clin Nutr* 1994 ; 59 : 1060-8.

• Nagata C, Takatsuka N, Inaba S, Kawakami N, Shimizu H. Effect of soymilk consumption on serum estrogen concentrations in premenopausal Japanese women. *J Natl Cancer Inst* 1998 ; 90 : 1830-5.

• Negri E, La Vecchia C, Franceschi S, *et al*. Vegetable and fruit consumption and cancer risk. *Int J Cancer* 1991 ; 48 : 350-4.

• Negri E, La Vecchia C, Franceschi S, D'Avanzo B, Talamini R, Parpinel M, Ferraroni M, Filiberti R, Montella M, Falcini F, Conti E, Decarli A. Intake of selected micronutrients and the risk of breast cancer. *Int J Cancer* 1996-a ; 65 : 140-4.

• Negri E, La Vecchia C, Franceschi S, Levi F, Parazzini F. Intake of selected micronutrients and the risk of endometrial carcinoma. *Cancer* 1996-b ; 77 : 917-23.

• Newcomb PA, Klein R, Klein BEK, Haffner S, Mares-Perlman J, Cruickshanks KJ, Marcus PM. Association of dietary and life-style factors with sex hormones in postmenopausal women. *Epidemiology* 1995 ; 6 : 318-21.

• Nomura AM, Kolonel LN. Prostate cancer : a current perspective. *Epidemiol Rev* 1991 ; 13 : 200-27.

• Noroozi M, Angerson WJ, Lean MEJ. Effects of flavonoids and vitamin C on oxidative DNA damage to human lymphocytes. *Am J Clin Nutr* 1998 ; 67 : 1210-8.

• Nyberg F, Agrenius V, Svartengren K, Svensson C, Pershagen. Dietary factors and risk of lung cancer in never-smokers. *Int J Cancer* 1998 ; 78 : 430-6.

• Nyyssonen K, Parviainen MT, Salonen R, Tuomilehto J, Salonen JT. Vitamin C deficiency and risk of myocardial infarction : prospective population study of men from Eastern Finland. *Br Med J* 1997 ; 314 : 634-8.

• Ocke MC, Bueno-de-Mesquita B, Feskens EJM, Van Staveren WA, Kroumhout D. Repeated measurements of vegetables, fruits, beta-carotene, and vitamins C and E in relation to lung cancer. *Am J Epidemiol* 1997 ; 145 : 358-65.

- Omenn GS, Goodman GE, Thornquist MD, *et al.* Risk factors for lung cancer and for intervention effects in CARET, the beta-carotene and retinol efficacy trial. *J Natl Cancer Inst* 1996 ; 88 : 1550-9.

- Pietinen P, Rimm EB, Korhonen P, Hartman AM, Willett WC, Albanes D, Virtamo J. Intake of dietary fiber and risk of coronary heart disease in a cohort of finnish men. The ATBC cancer prevention study. *Circulation* 1996 ; 94 : 2720-7.

- Potischman N, Swanson CA, Coates RJ, Gammon MD, Brogan DR, Curtis J, Brinton LA. Intake of food groups and associated micronutrients in relation to risk of early-stage breast cancer. *Int J Cancer* 1999 ; 82 : 315-21.

- Potter JD, *et al.* Colon cancer : a review of the epidemiology. *Epidemiol Rev* 1993 ; 15 : 499-545.

- Potter JD, *et al.* Vegetable and fruit consumption and adenomatous polyps. The University of Minnesota Cancer Prevention Unit Case Control Study. *Proc AACR* 1995 ; 36 : 1702.

- Rapola JM, Virtamo J, Ripatti S, Huttunen JK, Albanes D, Taylor PR, Heinonen OP. Randomised trial of alpha-tocopherol and beta-carotene supplements on incidence of major coronary events in men with previous myocardial infarction. *Lancet* 1997 ; 349 : 1715-20.

- Rasmussen O, Lauszus FF, Christiansen C, *et al.* Differential effects of saturated and monounsaturated fat on blood glucose and insulin responses in subjects with NIDD. *Am J Clin Nutr* 1996 ; 63 : 249-53.

- Reaven PD, Khouw A, Beltz WF, Parthasarathy S, Witzum JJ. Effect of dietary antioxidant combinations in human. *Arterioscler Thromb* 1993 ; 13 : 590-600.

- Rehm JT, Bondy SJ, Sempos CT, Vuong CV. Alcohol consumption and coronary heart disease morbidity and mortality. *Am J Epidemiol* 1997 ; 146 : 495-501.

- Renaud S, de Lorgeril M. Wine, alcohol, platelets and the French paradox or coronary disease. *Lancet* 1979 ; 1 : 1017-20.

- Richardson S, de Vincenzi I, Pujol H, Gerber M. Alcohol consumption in a case-control study of breast cancer in Southern France. *Int J Cancer* 1989 ; 44 : 84-9.

- Richardson S, Gerber M, Cenée S. The role of fat, animal protein and vitamin consumption in breast cancer. A case-control study in Southern France. *Int J Cancer* 1991 ; 48 : 1-9.

- Rimm EB, *et al.* Vegetable, fruit, and cereal fiber intake and risk of coronary heart disease among men. *JAMA* 1996 ; 275 : 447-51.

- Rimm EB, Willett WC, Sampson L, Colditz GA, Manson JE, Hennekens C, Stampfer MJ. Folate and vitamin B6 from diet and supplements in relation to risk of coronary heart disease among women. *JAMA* 1998 ; 279 : 359-64.

- Rimm EB, Stampfer MJ, Ascherio A, Giovanucci E, Colditz GA, Willett WC. Vitamin E consumption and risk of coronary heart disease in men. *N Engl J Med* 1993 ; 328 : 1450-6.

- Rohan TE, McMichael AJ, Baghurst PA. A population-based case-control study of diet and breast cancer in Australia. *Am J Epidemiol* 1988 ; 128 : 478-89.

- Romieu I, Meneses F, Ramirez M, Ruiz S, Perez Padilla R, Sienra JJ, Gerber M, Grievink L, Dekker R, Walda I, Brunekref B. Antioxidant supplementation and respiratory functions among workers exposed to high levels of ozone. *Am J Resp Crit Care Med* 1998 ; 158 : 226-32.

- Rouanet JM, Laurent C, Besançon P. Rice bran and wheat bran : selective effect on plasma and liver cholesterol in high-cholesterol fed rats. *Food Chemistry* 1993 ; 47 : 67-71.

- Sachs FM, *et al.* Effects of ingestion of meat on plasma cholesterol of vegetarians. *JAMA* 1981 ; 246 : 640-4.

- Saintot M, Astre C, Pujol H, Gerber M. Tumor Progression and Oxidant-Antioxidant Status. *Carcinogenesis* 1996 ; 17 : 1267-71.

- Salonen JT, *et al.* High stored iron levels are associated with excess risk of myocardial infarction in Eastern Finnish men. *Circulation* 1992 ; 86 : 803-11.

- Sandker GW, Kromhout D, Aravanis C, *et al.* Serum cholesteryl ester fatty acids and their relation with serum lipids in elderly men in Crete and the Netherlands. *Eur J Clin Nutr* 1993 ; 47 : 201-8.

- Scali J, Richard A, Gerber M. Diet profiles in a population sample from Mediterranean Southern France. *Public Heath Nutrition* 2001 (in press).

- Schorah CJ, Devitt H, Lucock M, Dowell AC. The responsiveness of plasma homocysteine to small increases in dietary folic acid : a primary care study. *Eur J Clin Nutr* 1998 ; 52 : 407-11.

- Setchell KDR. Phyto-oestrogens : the chemistry, physiology and implications for human health of soy isoflavones. *Am J Clin Nutr* 1968 ; 68(S) : 1333S-46S.

- Shikany JM, Witte JS, Henning SM, Swendseid ME, Bird CL, Frankl HD, Lee ER, Haile RW. Plasma carotenoids and the prevalence of adenomatous polyps of the distal colon and rectum. *Am J Epidemiol* 1997 ; 145 : 552-7.

- Silverman DT, Brown LM, Hoover RN, *et al.* Alcohol and pancreatic cancer in Blacks and Whites in the United States. *Cancer Res* 1995 ; 55 : 4899-905.

- Simopoulos A, Salem N Jr. Purslane : a terrestrial source of omega-3 fatty acids. *N Engl J Med* 1986 ; 315 : 833-5.

- Slattery ML, Caan BJ, Berry TD, Coates A, Duncan D, Edwards SL. Dietary energy sources and colon cancer risks. *Am J Epidemiol* 1997 ; 145 : 199-210.

- Stampfer MJ, Hennekens CH, Manson JE, *et al.* A prospective study of vitamin E consumption and risk of coronary heart disease in women. *N Engl J Med* 1993 ; 328 : 1444-9.

- Stephens NG, Parsons A, Schofield PM, Kelly F, Cheeseman K, Mitchinson MJ, Brown MJ. Randomised controlled trial of vitamin E in patients with coronary disease : Cambridge Heart Antioxidant Study (CHAOS). *Lancet* 1996 ; 347 : 781-6.

- Stoll BA. Breast cancer : further metabolic-endocrine risk markers ? *Br J Cancer* 1997 ; 76 : 1652-4.

- Suschetet M. Microconstituants végétaux présumés protecteurs. In : Riboli E, *et al.*, eds. *Alimentation et cancer*. Paris : Tec Doc, Lavoisier, 1996 : 459-508.

- Swain JF, Rouse IL, Curley CB, Sacks FM. Comparison of the effects of oat bran and low-fiber wheat on serum lipoprotein levels and blood pressure. *N Engl J Med* 1990 ; 322 : 147-52.

- Talamini R, La Vecchia C, Decarli A. Social factors, diet and breast cancer in a Northern Italian population. *Br J Cancer* 1984 ; 49 : 723-9.

- The alpha-tocopherol, beta-carotene cancer prevention study group. The effect of vitamin E and beta carotene on the incidence of lung cancer and other cancers in male smokers. *N Engl J Med* 1994 ; 330 : 1029-35.

- Thompson LU, *et al.* Influence of flaxseed and lignan on colon carcinogenesis. The role of lignans and oil in flaxseed on mammary tumorigenesis. *Proc AACR* 1995 ; 36 : 675-8.

- Thun MJ, Peto R, Lopez AK, Monaco JH, Henley J, Heath CW, Doll R. Alcohol consumption and mortality among middle-aged and elderly US adults. *N Engl J Med* 1997 ; 337 : 1705-14.

- Todd S, Woodward M, Tunstall-Pedoe H, Bolton-Smith C. Dietary antioxidant vitamins and fiber in the etiology of cardiovascular disease and all-causes mortality : results from the Scottish Heart Health Study. *Am J Epidemiol* 1999 ; 150 : 1073-80.

- Toniolo P, Riboli E, Protta F, *et al.* Calorie-providing nutriments and risk of breast cancer. *J Natl Cancer Inst* 1989 ; 81 : 278-86.

- Trichopoulou A, Katsouyanni K, Stuver S, *et al.* Consumption of olive oil and specific food groups in relation to breast cancer risk in Greece. *J Natl Cancer Inst* 1995 ; 87 : 110-5.

- Tzonou A, Lagiou P, Trichopoulou A, Tsoutsos V, Trichopoulos D. Dietary iron and coronary heart disease risk : a study from Greece. *Am J Epidemiol* 1998 ; 147 : 161-6.

- Van den Brandt P, Van't Veer P, Goldbohm RA, *et al.* A prospective cohort study on dietary fat and the risk of postmenopausal breast cancer. *Cancer Res* 1993 ; 53 : 75-82.

- Van't Veer P, Dekker JM, Lamers JW, *et al.* Consumption of fermented milk products and breast cancer : a case-control study in the Netherlands. *Cancer Res* 1989 ; 49 : 4020-3.

- Van't Veer P, Van Leer EM, Rietdijk A, *et al.* Combination of dietary factors in relation to breast-cancer occurence. *Int J Cancer* 1991 ; 47 : 649-53.

• Van't Veer P, Strain JJ, Fernandez-Crehuet J, Martin BC, Thamm M, Kardinaal AF, Kohlmeier L, Huttunen JF, Martin-Moreno JM, Kok FJ. Tissue antioxidants and postmenopausal breast cancer : the European Community Multicentre Study on Antioxidants, Myocardial Infarction, and Cancer of the Breast (EURAMIC). *Cancer Epidemiol Biom Prev* 1996 ; 5 : 441-7.

• Verhoeven DTH, Assen N, Goldbohm RA, Dorant E, Van'T Veer P, Sturmans F, Hermus RJJ, Van Den Brandt PA. Vitamins C and E, retinol, beta-carotene and dietary fibre in relation to breast cancer risk : a prospective cohort study. *Br J Cancer* 1997 ; 75 : 149-55.

• Visioli F, Galli C. The effect of minor constituents of olive oil on cardiovascular disease : new findings. *Nutr Rev* 1998 ; 56 : 142-7.

• Wahlqvist ML, Wattanapenpaiboon N, Macrae FA. Changes in serum carotenoids in subjects with colo-rectal adenomas after 24 months of beta-carotene supplementation. *Am J Clin Nutr* 1998 ; 90 : 583-612.

• Willett WC, Stampfer MJ, Colditz GA, Rosner BA, Speizer FE. Relation of meat, fat, and fiber, intake to the risk of colon cancer in a prospective study among women. *N Engl J Med* 1990 ; 323 : 1664-72.

• Willet WC, Hunter DJ, Stampfer MJ, et al. Dietary fat and fiber in relation to risk of breast cancer : an eight year follow-up. *JAMA* 1992 ; 268 : 2037-44.

• Wiseman H. The bioavailability of non-nutrient plant factors : dietary flavonoids and phyto-oestrogens. *Proc Nutr Soc* 1999 ; 58 : 139-46.

• Witte JS, Longnecker MP, Bird CL, Lee ER, Frankl HD, Haile RW. Relation of vegetable, fruit, and grain consumption to colorectal adenomatous polyps. *Am J Epidemiol* 1996 ; 144 : 1015-25.

• Wolk A, Bergstrom R, Hunter D, Willett W, Ljung H, Holmberg L, Bergkvist L, Bruce A, Adami HO. A prospective study of association of monounsaturated fat and other types of fat with risk of breast cancer. *Arch Intern Med* 1998 ; 158 : 41-5.

• Wolk A, Mason JA, Stampfer MJ, Colditz GA, Hu FB, Speizer FE, Hennekens CH, Willett. Long-term intake of dietary fiber and decreased risk of coronary heart disease amon women. *JAMA* 1999 ; 281 : 1998-2004.

• Yong LC, Brown CC, Schatzkin A, Dresser CM, Slesinski MJ, Cox CS, Taylor PR. Intake of vitamins E, C, and A and risk of lung cancer. The NHANES I epidemiologic follow up study. *Am J Epidemiol* 1997 ; 146 : 231-43.

• Yu S, Derr J, Etherton TD, Kris-Etherton PM. Plasma-cholesterol-predictive equations demonstrate that stearic acid id neutral and monounsaturated fatty acids are hypocholesterolemic. *Am J Clin Nutr* 1995 ; 61 : 1129-39.

• Yu SZ, Lu RF, Xu DD, et al. A case-control study of dietary and non dietary risk factors for breast cancer in Shangaï. *Cancer Res* 1990 ; 50 : 5017-21.

• Zhang S, Tang G, Russell RM, Mayzel KA, Stampfer MJ, Willett WC, Hunter DJ. Measurement of retinoids and carotenoids in breast adipose tissue and a comparison of concentrations in breast cancer cases and control subjects. *Am J Clin Nutr* 1997 ; 66 : 626-32.

• Zhang S, Hunter DJ, Hankinson SE, Giovannucci EL, Rosner BA, Colditz GA, Speizer FE, Willett WC. A prospective study of folate intake and the risk of breast cancer. *JAMA* 1999 ; 281(17) : 1632-7.

• Nyyssonen K, Parviainen MT, Salonen R, Tuomilehto J, Salonen JT. Vitamen C deficiency and risk of myocardial infarction: prospective population study of men from eastern Finland. *Br Med J* 1997; 314: 634-8.

• Scali J, Richard A, Gerber M. Diet profiles in a population sample from Mediterranean Southern France. *Public Health Nutrition* 2001 (in press).

Nutritional contribution of food in the Mediterranean consumption model

Olive oil, olive oil by-products and olive fruit: current data and developments concerning the food and health relationship

Claude-Louis Léger, Bernard Descomps

The consumption of olives and olive oil is one of the major characteristics of the Mediterranean type diet. Epidemiological data and nutritional interventions indicate that some of the "health benefit" attributed to this type of food can be attributed to olive oil consumption (*see chapter* "Health benefits of the Mediterranean consumption model"). This recent idea, as well as the organoleptic qualities of products (appearance of controlled origin denominations) give rise to increased interest in the culture of the olive tree in Southern Europe, as well as in the Languedoc-Roussillon and Provence-Alpes-Côte d'Azur in France. The following report tries to differentiate between what is known and possible in terms of health benefit due to olive oil consumption: the role of oleic acid intake (fatty acid characteristic of olive oil) and the possible contribution of polyphenols, as non-glyceride minor components (whose biological activity is not limited to an anti-oxidant effect).

Olive undoubtedly benefits from a positive image in public opinion with respect to health, thus presenting a very strong opposition to the generally negative image given by dietary lipids (fats!). In order to be convinced it suffices to observe the increase in consumption:

– in France: + 78% between 1984 and 1996 (Barsacq, 1997);

– in the world: + 23% from 1990 to 1997 for all the countries disposing of consumption statistics, + 67% when only the olive oil producing countries are considered (Luchetti, 1997).

The United States, first olive oil importing country, is characterized by a type consumption that evolutes as that of a non-producing country, since olive oil consumption (mainly a mixture of extra virgin olive oil and refined olive oil) has increased by 20%, while the total oil consumption by the populations has decreased by 20% (Haumann, 1996).

In general, countries with the lowest consumption a few years ago, or that did not reach a measurable level of consumption, have progressed the most. This is particularly true for Northern European countries where consumption has been multiplied by three in the last ten years (Barsac, 1997).

The olive oil craze has also been illustrated by the launching of a genetic improvement programme that has resulted in the commercialization of oleisol, *i.e.* a sunflower oil with a fatty acid composition that resembles that of olive oil.

This opinion movement is comparable and simultaneous to that which recognizes a beneficial role in terms of health for the Mediterranean diet. Thus reputation of olive oil is not unfounded.

EPIDEMIOLOGICAL STUDIES:
PIONEER STUDIES ON THE MEDITERRANEAN DIET

The broad outline has been mentioned in the first chapter of this work. We will only develop the major stages concerning cardiovascular diseases.

Ancel Keys was the first to observe in the 1950s that Mediterranean populations presented a lower cardiovascular morbidity and mortality than Western populations (especially Northern Europe and the United States). He also observed, and thus confirmed previous observations, that the populations with the highest cardiovascular risk were characterized by high blood cholesterol levels (Keys, 1957).

Many works and an abundant literature have since been dedicated to the relationship between blood cholesterol levels and cardiovascular risk. They definitively established that an increase in blood (or plasma) cholesterol levels was a marker and a major risk factor for cardiovascular diseases. However, the majority of the studies concluded to the absence of relationship between dietary cholesterol consumed and cardiovascular risk. Moreover, it is established today that within the limits of a normal diet, dietary cholesterol has little influence on blood cholesterol levels (Connor and Connor, 1995).

The most innovative result of the studies carried out at the end of the 1950s by A. Keys, first published in 1957 (Anderson *et al.*, 1957), was to demonstrate that an increase in total blood cholesterol and low density lipoproteins cholesterol or LDL was directly related to lipid rich food intake.

The Seven Country Study (Finland, United States, Netherlands, Italy, Croatia, Serbia, Greece and Japan) started in the beginning of the 1960s, and continued over more than twenty years, resulting in numerous publications, largely confirmed these results. The first publications established that the Mediterranean diet provided in the 1950s less than half the amount of lipids (in energy) than the North American diet (Keys *et al.*, 1954). However a substantial detail could be given: only a portion of the lipids consumed was important, as only the saturated lipids (fatty acids without double bond or unsaturation) were directly correlated to cholesterolemia. Mediterranean diet provided small amounts of saturated fatty acids, generally less than half that of the Northern European countries and the United States. Olive oil, low in saturated fatty acids, could represent up to 80% of the lipid intake in the diet of some Mediterranean countries, when these observations were made. The ratio between monounsaturated (a single double bond or unsaturation) and saturated fatty acids (an indicator of consumption of olive oil relative to total fat consumption) gave a better account of the variability in cardiovascular mortality risks (Keys *et al.*, 1986).

THE EFFECT OF THE DRIFT IN CONSUMPTION

The main result of the Seven Country Study is the fact that thanks to it we have convincing epidemiological arguments of a relationship between the nature of dietary fat, cholesterolemia and cardiovascular risk (Kromhout *et al.*, 1986). During the study, a positive drift in meat and milk consumption was observed, which was accompanied of an increase in cardiovascular risk.

OLIVE OIL ACTIVE COMPONENTS IN TERMS OF HEALTH

It is necessary to separate the solidly acquired knowledge, from that which requires additional comments. We must make a distinction between the properties of olive oil due to the fatty acid fraction from those that cannot be attributed, in the current state of knowledge, to a specific fraction of the oil: fatty acid fraction, phenolic fraction or other non-glyceride fractions.

PREVENTIVE ROLE WITH RESPECT TO CARDIOVASCULAR DISEASES ATTRIBUTABLE TO OLEIC ACID

Extra virgin olive oil contains 53 to 80% of oleic acid (the most representative of the mono-unsaturated acids: a single double bond), *versus* 3 to 20% of linoleic acid (two double bonds), and 10 to 20% of saturated acids (mostly palmitic acid).

The latter is principally situated in the external position (sn-1/sn-3) of a triglyceride molecule (less than 10% of palmitic acid is in sn-2 position, *versus* approximately 70% of linoleic acid and 50% of oleic acid).

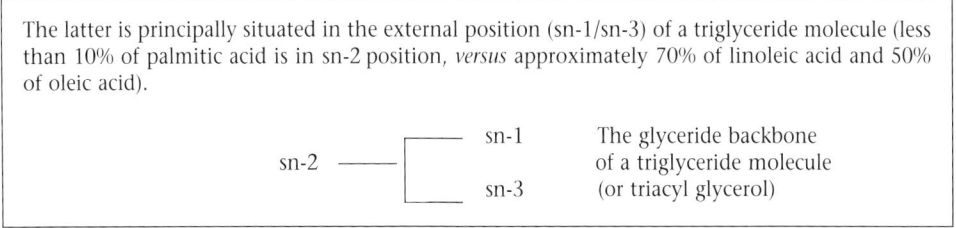

Today it is currently admitted that, compared to saturated fatty acids, oleic acid is a hypo-cholesterolemic agent. The groups of Grundy, Mensink and Katan (Grundy, 1986); Mattson, Grundy, 1985; Mensink and Katan, 1987; Garg *et al.*, 1988; Mensink *et al.*, 1989) had already suggested that the replacement of saturated fats with mono-unsaturated fats led to a reduction in total plasma cholesterol and low density lipoprotein cholesterol (or "bad cholesterol"), at least equal to that obtained by a simple reduced intake of saturated fats.

This was confirmed by Ginsberg *et al.* (1990) in a study on 36 healthy subjects who received for 10 weeks diets providing the following:

– 38% of lipids with 18/10/10 saturated fatty acids (SFA), mono-unsaturated fatty acids (MUFA) and poly-unsaturated fatty acids (PUFA- several double bonds or unsaturations), respectively;

– or 30% of lipids with 10/10/10 of the three types of fatty acids;

– or 38% of lipids with 10/18/10 SFA, MUFA and PUFA.

It was possible to determine (Ginsberg *et al.*, 1990; Mensink and Katan, 1989; Berry *et al.*, 1991) that the decrease in total plasma cholesterol was due to a reduction in the cholesterol transported by LDL. The hypocholesterolemic effect of oleic acid was comparable to that of linoleic acid, when the effect of saturated fatty acids was taken as the reference. Oleic acid generally did not show an effect on HDL cholesterol (high density lipoprotein cholesterol). HDL cholesterol is commonly considered as "good cholesterol" as it represents an elimination route. However, it has also been mentioned that the consumption of oleic acid does not modify or may increase the plasma level of HDL cholesterol (Mattson and Grundy, 1985; Mensink and Katan, 1987) while linoleic acid rich food intake where shown to have the inverse effect (Mattson and Grundy, 1985). Given the relationship between an increase in HDL cholesterol and a decrease in cardiovascular risk (Framingham Study; Wilson *et al.*, 1988), this oleic acid effect may be considered as a protective effect, an interesting one as it opposes that of the unsaturated fatty acid most preponderant in commonly used cooking oils (sunflower, corn, soy).

A recent study confirms the positive role of oleic acid in cardiovascular prevention in a population of 80,000 women in the Nurses' Health Study (Hu, 1997) (Massachusetts), irrespective of the dietary origin of this acid. This role could be explained by the greater capacity of cholesterol to be bound by HDL from persons who consume olive oil, than by HDL from persons who consume polyunsaturated oils (Esteva *et al.*, 1986).

OLEIC ACID AND THE DECREASE IN LDL OXIDATION

It was finally clearly demonstrated in animals that oleic acid, with low oxidation potential due to its monounsaturation, lowers the oxidation potential of LDL when it substitutes a polyunsaturated fatty acid in conditions of energy intake between 20 and 30% of total energy (Parthasarathy *et al.*, 1990; Wiseman *et al.*, 1996; Scaccini *et al.*, 1992). In humans, an olive oil supplementation of 50 g/day for a week significantly reduces the oxidation potential of LDL and their incorporation by a macrophage strain (Aviram and Eias, 1993), while oleic acid incubated in the presence of LDL inhibits LDL oxidation in a dose-dependent manner. The multiple roles played by oxidized forms of LDL in the atherogenic process are known, in particular their capacity to incorporate themselves in a special type of white blood cells, *i.e.* the macrophages (cells in charge of phagocytosing bacteria) that form "foam" cells and lipid strakes characteristic of the first clinical stage of atheroma (Parthasaraty and Rankin, 1992). Therefore, it is possible to think that a better antioxidant protection of LDL due to oleic acid enrichment supports an improved protection against atherosclerosis.

OLIVE OIL AND THE DIGESTIVE APPARATUS

This subject was thoroughly treated by Charbonnier, 1996. It will be simply reminded here that extra virgin olive oil is considered by gastro-enterologists as an agent of choice in the contraction of the gall bladder. Therefore, it is a cholagogue that cannot be replaced in this role by any other cooking oil. This property is not modified after heating at 200 °C for 3 hours. Furthermore, olive oil seems to be the oil that slows down gastric evacuation least, and one of those with the most effective intestinal absorption (all studies included, its digestibility is greater than 94%).

OLIVE OIL AND CANCER

The data available today are mainly epidemiological; they were analysed in the first chapter of this book, and the general aspects of the relationships between dietary lipids and the risk of cancer were the subjects of a recent editorial (Wisout, 1999).

Two studies carried out in Southern European countries (Trichopoulou *et al.*, 1994; Martine Moreno *et al.*, 1994; Franceschi *et al.*, 1996) indicate that a decrease in the risk of breast cancer is associated with a major consumption of olive oil. It is interesting to relate these data to another result of a large study carried out in Northern Europe on a population of 61,000 Swedish women (Wolk *et al.*, 1998) which mentions a decrease in breast cancer associated with a high consumption of mono-unsaturated fatty acids. Thus, it could be thought that the beneficial effect can be attributed to oleic acid itself, as in Northern Europe olive oil consumption is low. However, the results of the Swedish study were qualified and the origin of the monounsaturated fatty acids was not specified.

Drawing a conclusion requires to be carefull in this topic for several reasons:

– to attribute to oleic acid the risk modifications observed, it is essentiall to know what is provided by its own high consumption and what is provided by the associated consumption of polyphenols, as well as what is the consequence of the substitution of this acid by other acids in particular linoleic acid whose consumption decreases concomitantly when that of oleic acid increases;

– a majority of epidemiological studies seem to indicate that an increase in the risk of certain cancers is associated with an increase in lipid consumption, all the results are not in accordance;

– it remains difficult to distinguish what belongs to an increase in lipid dietary intake, especially the nature of the constitutive fatty acids, and what is due to excess calories, low physical activity and excess weight that frequently accompanies the over-consumption of fatty acids.

PHENOLIC COMPOUNDS IN OLIVE OIL, OLIVES AND OLIVE OIL WASTEWATERS

Apart from the glyceride fraction, extra virgin olive oil contains a non-glyceride fraction with the characteristics shown in *Table I*. It is mostly made up of hydrocarbons (squalene, a metabolic cholesterol precursor), but also contains sterols (substances related to cholesterol), triterpenic alcohols, as well as, in approximately equivalent amounts, tochopherols (vitamin E and derivatives) and phenolic compounds (Uzzan, 1992; Tsimidou *et al.*, 1992; Forcadell *et al.*, 1987; Akabi *et al.*, 1993), some of which are comparable to those found in wine.

Table I. Composition of the non-glyceride fraction of the extra virgin olive oil

Oil content:	0.4-0.8% including:	
	• Hydrocarbons	including squalene 300-700 mg/100 g
	• Sterols	including β-sitosterol 70-90 mg/100 g
	• Triterpenic alcohols	100-300 mg/100 g
	• Tocopherols	7-15 mg/100 g
	α-tocopherols	4-13 mg/100 g
	β-tocopherols	1-2 mg/100 g
	• Phenolic compounds	2-50 mg/100 g
	hydroxytyrosol	0.01-1 mg/100 g

It has been reported that the ingestion of squalene at a dose of 1 g/day, equivalent to the consumption of 100 g of olive oil for the most squalene-rich oils, increased the atherogenic forms of plasma cholesterol transport, but 0.5 g/day of squalene administered afterwards normalises plasma sterols (Miettinene and Vanhanen, 1994). Phytosterols (plant sterols), including the most abundant β-sitosterol, are also the subject of research. Olive oil contains ten to twenty times less than corn oil. This has been partly related to discrepancies between the effects of these oils on circulating cholesterol and triglycerides (Howell *et al.*, 1998).

We will discuss here the phenolic compounds which are specific to olive oil, which are not common to any other common cooking oil and are of organoleptic and nutritional interest.

Olive present variable polyphenol contents. Basically it depends on the variety and the degree of maturity on harvest (Vazquez Roncero, 1978, Amiot *et al.*, 1986, 1988). The values were between 1 and 10 g/kg of olives in a recent study on four different varieties from Spain, Italy, Portugal and France (Vincieri *et al.*, personal communication), but higher contents have been reported (Vazquez Roncero, 1978). Polyphenol content in olive oil depends not only on the variety, maturity of the fruits, and cultivation conditions, but also on the technological processes employed to separate the aqueous phase (vegetable olive oil wastewaters (OOWW)) from the oil phase (olive oil, strictly speaking). It varies from 100 mg to 1 g/kg for olive oil and 40 mg to 7 g/l for OOWW (Perrin, 1992). It is generally estimated that 1 kg of olives provides 0.5 to 1 l of OOWW. However, certain separation processes lower OOWW volume produced and thus concentrate the polyphenols, both in OOWW and oil. The high polyphenol content of

OOWW, greater than that of the oil phase, results from amphiphilic properties, but mainly hydrophilic, of these compounds. Since a fraction of these polyphenols is consumed when black olives are themselves consumed, it can be expected that the inconvenient "pollutant" can be transformed in an advantage, on condition to take care of the OOWW as soon as they come out of the centrifuge. Studies are currently in progress to valorise the vegetable water polyphenols as "natural antioxidants" that may be used in various agro-food fields.

Oleuropein, a phenolic secoiridoid, is the main phenolic compound in olives, responsible for the fruit's bitterness. During the technological processes, this compound undergoes chemical transformations (hydrolysis and oxidations). In olive oil phenolic compounds such as hydroxycinnamic esters are found. These compounds can participate in the stability of the oil according to the following mechanisms: free radical scavengers, protectors of other antioxidant molecules and metal chelators, as metals are excellent catalysts of oxidations. If these compounds have antioxidant properties that have been demonstrated *in vivo*, they may also have a protective effect with respect to LDL oxidation, of which we have already mentioned the crucial role in developing atheromatous lesions. Real biological effects of these molecules depend on their absorption and metabolism. Few studies have been dedicated to their bioavailability so far. However, a certain number of *in vitro* data are already available.

The following is a more detailed description of the phenolic compounds (*see technical information*: "Polyphenols: an introduction"):

– phenolic alcohols: tyrosol and hydroxytyrosol,

– free phenolic acids belonging to the benzoic series: protocatechuic, gallic, vanillic, and syringic acids, or to the cinnamic series: p-coumaric, caffeic and sinapic acids,

– caffeic acid (verbascoside) or elenolic acid (oleuropein glycosylated or not, mainly responsible for bitterness) esterified by hydroxytyrosol,

– flavonoids: flavones (luteolin) and flavonols (quercetin and kaemferol glycosylated or not).

It has already been mentioned that the phenolic compound content of olives depends on the degree of maturity and variety. This is a real issue randering the identification of varieties and the control of their specificity difficult. However, the genotype diversity of olive tree is at the same time a wealth that should be preserved for the potentially interesting products it may provide.

The genetic diversity of olive tree is considerable. It is marked through the morphology and phenology of the trees, helping to list and manage the collections. However, it is influenced by environmental effects which perturb its expression, leading to erroneous evaluation. The molecular diversity observed by gene analysis is by contrast independent of the environment. It can be used for variety identification, clonal diversity and to determine the degree of relatedness of cultivars. It allows the detection of homonymies (same name for different clones) and synonymies (different names for the same clone). In the lineage of one crossing of two varieties, this leads to the construction of a genetic map to establish the relationship between the markers and the segregation characters. Therefore, it is an essential complement for managing collections and improving varieties.

Genetic studies have shown that the Mediterranean olive tree has several origins in other European varieties. Their diversity, as well as their adaptation to very different environments, make them a precious but insufficiently studied genetic resource. Few hybridization experiments have been carried out. Can these species provide olive tree with the characteristics it lacks? In any case, marking the characters followed by assisted selection should result in the resistance to disease or environmental factors, and the improved control of the quality of the fatty acid and polyphenol composition.

As a general rule, the most abundant phenolic compounds are oleuropein, its glycosylated derivatives and its hydrolysis products. Certain varieties may also be rich in flavonoids. Olive oil contains five major compounds: tyrosol, hydroxytyrosol, p-hydroxyphenylacetic acid, homovanillic acid and caffeic acid *(Table II)*. The presence of 3,4-dihydroxy-phenylacetic acid is sometimes reported. The composition of OOWW is characterized mainly by the presence of elenolic acid, a oleuropein hydrolysis product, and in addition of the tyrosol/hydroxytyrosol couple (Vincieri *et al.*, unpublished data).

Table II. Phenolic compounds in four olive oil varieties in mg/kg (Akasbi *et al*, 1993)

Source	OH-tyrosol	Tyrosol	p-OH-phenylacetic acid	Homovanillic acid	Caffeic acid
Gondola	0.18 ± 0.007	9.62 ± 1.34	2.79 ± 0.30	0.23 ± 0.005	0.030 ± 0.01
Olio Sasso	0.19 ± 0.015	0.75 ± 0.29	0.19 ± 0.11	0.03 ± 0.008	0.014 ± 0.001
Fillipo Berio	0.57 ± 0.035	2.36 ± 0.45	0.31 ± 0.006	0.03 ± 0.002	nd[a]
Marca Il Duomo	0.74 ± 0.170	2.61 ± 1.25	1.73 ± 0.06	0.14 ± 0.026	nd[a]

[a] Not detected.

BIOLOGICAL PROPERTIES OF POLYPHENOLS

The effects of olive oil can only be attributed to the entire oil, in the current state of knowledge, which means that a possible intervention of the non-glyceride fraction of the oil may be suspected. Among these effects the following should be mentioned: decrease in blood pressure in hyperlipidemic patients (Nydahl *et al.*, 1994); platelet aggregation (Vicario *et al.*, 1998), plasma fibrinogen (Lopez-Segura, 1996), or even increase in bone density (Laval-Jeantet, 1983). Some biological properties of phenolic compounds are already reported in *Table III*.

ANTIOXIDANT PROPERTIES OF POLYPHENOLS

They have an antioxidant activity which varies as a function of their structure. Hydroxytyrosol is well-known for the "anti-peroxide" protection it provides to extra virgin olive oil (Perrin, 1992). It is also the most rapidly degraded during olive oil autoxidation (Chimi *et al.*, 1990). In this type of protection, only the ortho-diphenolic compounds were found to be active.

Table III. Biological effects of phenolic compounds present in olives

Family of compounds	Compounds	Biological properties
All families	Separately or in natural mixture (OOWW)	• Antioxidants[a] (Visioli et al., 1995) • Free radical scavenger[a] (Perrin, 1992) • LDL cytotoxicity[b]
Phenolic acids	Caffeic acid	• Anti-AP-1[a] • Anti-5-LIPOX (Koshihara et al., 1984)
Phenolic alcohols	Hydroxytyrosol Hydroxytyrosol derivatives • verbascoside • oleuropein	• Anti-platelet aggregation (Petroni et al., 1995) • Inhibits 5 and 12-LIPOX (Kohyama et al., 1997) • Inhibits TXB_2 (Petroni et al., 1995) • Anti-PKC (Herbert et al., 1991) • Anti-aldose-reductase (Andary, 1993) • Anti-proliferator (Andary, 1993) • Immunomodulator (Andary, 1993) • Synthesis of NO (Visioli et al., 1998)
Flavonoids	Flavonols Flavones Rutin (deconjugated = quercetin) Luteolin, quercetin	• Antiviral (Selway, 1986) • Inhibit T4 de-iodination (especially luteolin) (Köhrle et al., 1986) • Immunostimulator in irradiated or burnt patients • Anti-5-LIPOX (Welton et al., 1986) • Anti-aldose-reductase (Chaudhry et al., 1983) • Anti-PKC (Middleton, Ferriola, 1988)

[a] See text for bibliographical reference.
[b] Consequence of LDL oxido-protection.

In vitro protection of LDL against oxidation by hydroxytyrosol or oxidized derivatives of oleuropein was demonstrated (Visioli et al., 1995). The oxidation of LDL in rabbits having received extra virgin olive oil enriched feed, was less than that of LDL from rabbits having received a feed enriched either in refined olive oil (without polyphenols), or in sunflower oil (oil with similar fatty acid composition, but deprived of polyphenols) (Wiseman et al., 1996).

Table IV presents the specific antioxidant activities (SAA) of several olive phenolic acids, measured in our laboratory (in press) during the *in vitro* oxidation of human LDL performed in the presence of molecular oxygen and an oxidation catalyst (Cu^{2+}) *(figure 1)*. The aim of such a study was to compare the anti-oxidant potential of each molecule in order to evaluate their possible intervention in the anti-oxidant protection of LDL, one of the consequences of which, as we have already mentioned above, is an increased protection against atherosclerosis. We confirm the low antioxidant potential of the monophenolic structure (for example p-coumaric acid) in comparison with the ortho-diphenol structure (caffeic acid). Most phenolic acids studied also have a SAA independent of the concentration tested. The benzoic series acids, gallic and protocatechuic, present a variable SAA, higher at the submicromolar concentrations, that are likely to be encountered in plasma after ingestion of food rich in polyphenols.

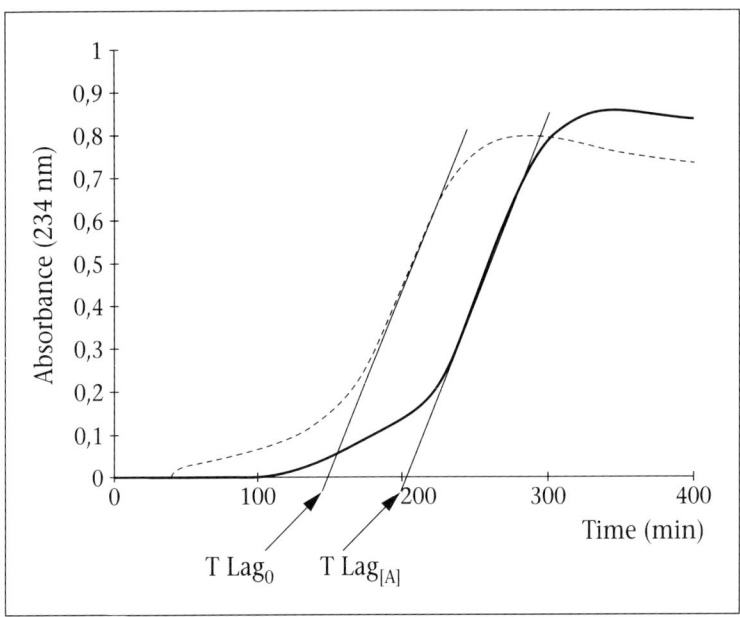

Figure 1. Method of calculation of specific antioxidant activity. The rate of conjugated diene production during LDL oxidation catalyzed by Cu^{2+} is represented under two conditions, with and without antioxidant. The lag time of the phenomenon in the absence of antioxidant, $T\ Lag_0$, is subtracted from the lag time in the presence of the concentration of an antioxidant A, $T\ Lag_{[A]}$ and [A] respectively. This difference value is plotted against increasing concentrations of A. The slope of the dose-response relationship is SAA.

Furthermore, it is well-known that the antioxidant activity of some substances with respect to LDL leads to the protection of the main antioxidant of this lipoprotein, vitamin E.

We were able to demonstrate that LDL protection by polyphenols present in olives and their by-products resulted in a decreased or a delayed production of lysophosphatidylcholine. This pro-inflammatory (and atherogenic) substance generally indicates the concomitant presence of oxidized phospholipid structurally and functionally related to PAF (a powerful pro-aggregatory factor) and involved in atherogenic process. This action means that polyphenols are potentially anti-arethomatous and anti-inflammatory substances.

In conclusion, extra virgin olive oil has two anti-oxidant characteristics:

– one "passive", due to the fatty acid it contains, mainly mono-unsaturated which cannot be oxidized easily,

– the other "active", due to the fact that it contains potentially active antioxidants.

Table IV. Specific antioxidant activity of different compounds or mixture of phenolic compounds

	Chemical formula	SAA[a] (AA Unit)	R[b]	p[c]	
Vegetable waters (extract)		7.2	0.964	< 1 %	n = 9
Red wine (extracts)		7.7	0.983	< 1 %	n = 7
p-coumaric acid	OH—⌬—CH=CH—COOH	0.5	0.684	< 1 %	n = 20
Ferulic acid	OH—⌬(CH$_3$O)—CH=CH—COOH	8.5	0.753	< 1 %	n = 20
Sinapic acid	OH—⌬(CH$_3$O)$_2$—CH=CH—COOH	47.4	0.896	< 1 %	n = 14
Caffeic acid	OH,OH—⌬—CH=CH—COOH	54.2	0.760	< 1 %	n = 24
Gallic acid	(OH)$_3$—⌬—COOH	from ≈ 750 to ≈ 10[d]			
Protocatechic acid	(OH)$_2$—⌬—COOH	from ≈ 1 000 to ≈ 10[d]			

[a] For the definition of unit, see figure 1.
[b] Coefficient of correlation of the dose-activity relationship.
[c] Statistical significance of the relationship.
[d] Submicromolar concentrations and micromolar and greater concentrations, respectively.

OTHER PROPERTIES OF POLYPHENOLS

Polyphenols present also other important biological properties.

Polyphenols, cell signalling and transcription factors

Two "general" properties could explain some specific effects: the anti-AP-1 and anti-PKC activities. The anti-AP-1 activity must be placed in a larger context, that of the effects of some antioxidants on at least two transcription factors sensitive to the redox state of the cell: AP-1 (for activating protein 1) and NFkappaB (NFκB) (for nuclear factor κB) (Chandan and Packer, 1996). This is a large domain of investigation that has been recently opened up, and is very promising for the genomic regulations it should lead to explain or find out. On the one hand, the binding sites of these two transcription factors are located in a promoter region of a great number of genes directly involved in the pathogenesis of diseases as diverse as atherosclerosis, diabetes, AIDS and cancer (Chandan and Packer, 1996). On the other hand, it is interesting to note that the AP1 transcription factor presents at least one binding site in the promoter region of the selenium-dependent glutathion peroxydase gene (Jornot, Jundo, 1997), an important antioxidant enzyme present in the cytoplasm of cells. This suggests the possibility of a potentialisation of cellular enzymatic defences by anti-oxidants.

In general, antioxidants (vitamin E, antioxidant catechols) suppress the DNA binding activity of NFκB (Suzuki and Packer, 1993 a and b), while the DNA binding activity of AP-1, as well as the mRNA expression of c-fos and c-jun (constitutive oncogenes of AP-1), responds positively (Choi and Moore, 1993). For example, a caffeic acid ester, more lipophilic than the free acid, specifically inhibits NFκB binding (Natarajan et al., 1996). We have demonstrated (unpublished result) that phenolic acids – the most active being caffeic acid – inhibit AP-1 activity in transfected MTLN cells expressing an enzymatic activity (luciferase) depending on the AP-1 binding site.

PKC (protein kinase C) is an ubiquitous transduction effector of numerous extra-cellular signals. In particular it intervenes upstream on the two mechanisms involved in inflammatory and atherogenic processes: vascular smooth muscle cell proliferation and production of superoxide anion by monocytes/macrophages. When an ear oedema is induced in mice using phorbol myristate acetate (PMA) – PKC specific pharmacological agonist – an inhibition of the inflammatory processes by catechol type phenolic acids (including caffeic acid and protocatechuic acid) is obtained (Fernandez et al., 1998). We showed that the polyphenolic fractions from OOWW are capable of scavenging the superoxide anion produced by a differentiated promonocyte cell line, and to strongly decrease the cellular production of superoxide in this PMA-stimulated cell line (Léger et al., 2000). Luteolin, a flavone present in olives and its by-products, is one of the more powerful PKC inhibitory flavonoids (Middleton and Ferriola, 1988).

Luteolin is also a powerful antithyroid agent, acting as an inhibitor of the enzymatic deiodination of low activity thyroxin T4 into tri-iodo-thyronine T3 (Koehrle et al., 1986), which is twenty times more active.

Effects mentioned in *Table III* probably play a key role in vascular pathologies: specifically, the anti-5-lipoxygenase action (thus anti-inflammatory) of caffeic acid and rutin, anti-aggregation and antithromboxane actions of hydroxytyrosol (thus antithrombotic and vasorelaxant) and the stimulating action on endothelial synthesis of nitrogen monoxide, a powerful vasorelaxant of the vascular wall.

The inhibition of aldose reductase by verbascoside and rutin could suggest a preventative role of olives and their by-products in diabetes-related cataracts. It seems that this possibility has not been explored in nutritional epidemiology.

Finally, a recent study opens new perspectives on the role of antioxidants in osteoporosis (Parhami *et al.*, 1997). Oxidized LDL seems to facilitate calcium storage in atherosclerotic vascular walls, however they block the differentiation of osteoblasts, which could explain the lack of bone calcification. Restoring bone calcium accretion by antioxidants could be envisaged. Is it this type of action – added to the oleic acid effect suggested up to now – that would be responsible for the correlation observed in 1984 by Laval-Jeantet *et al.* between an increase in bone density and an increase in olive oil consumption (Laval-Jeantet *et al.*, 194).

The biological activities of polyphenols which have just been reported as well as the routes to be explored involve the non glyceride fraction of extra virgin olive oil in highly relevant actions in terms of health and prevention. A clear demonstration of a real effect on health of the non-glyceride fraction remains necessary prior to envisaging an extensive use of the properties of these compounds in food and culinary products. Could olive itself be promoted, as a fruit, vegetable and oil as well, in dishes which are to a large extent to be (re-)invented?

REFERENCES

- Akasbi M, Shoeman DW, Csallany AS. High-performance liquid chromatography of selected phenolic compounds in olive oils. *J Am Oil Chem Soc* 1993 ; 70 : 368-70.

- Amiot MJ, Fleuriet A, Macheix JJ. Importance and evolution of phenolic compounds in olive during growth and maturation. *J Agric Food Chem* 1986 ; 34 : 823-6.

- Amiot MJ, Fleuriet A, Macheix JJ. Accumulation of oleuropein derivatives during olive maturation. *Phytochemistry* 1988 ; 28 : 67-9.

- Andary C. Caffeic acid glycoside esters and pharmacology. In : Scalbert A, ed. *Polyphenolic phenomena*. Paris : édition INRA, 1993 : 237-45.

- Anderson JT, Keys A, Grande F. Effects of different food fats on serum cholesterol concentrations. *Lancet* 1957 ; 1 : 787.

- Aviram M, Eias K. Dietary olive oil reduces low-density lipoprotein uptake by macrophages and decrease the susceptibility of the lipoprotein to undergo lipid peroxidation. *Ann Nutr Metab* 1993 ; 37 : 75-84.

- Barsacq JC. Le secteur de l'huile d'olive au sein de l'Union Européenne : situation et rôle de la Communauté. *OCL* 1997 ; 4 : 340-5.

- Berry EM, Eisenberg S, Haratz D, Friedlander Y, Norman Y, Kaufmann NA, Stein Y. Effects of diets rich in monounsaturated fatty acids on plasma lipoproteins – The Jerusalem Nutrition Study : high MUFAs *vs* high PUFAs. *Am J Clin Nutr* 1991 ; 53 : 899-907.

- Chandan KS, Packer L. Antioxidant and redox regulation of gene transcription. *FASEB J* 1996 ; 10 : 709-20.

- Charbonnier A. L'huile d'olive et l'appareil digestif. In : *L'huile d'olive : aliment-santé*. Paris : Frison-Roche, 1996 : 205-27.

- Chaudhry PS, Cabrera J, Juliani HR, Varma SD. Inhibition of human lens aldose reductase by flavonoids, sulindac and indomethacin. *Biochem Pharmacol* 1983 ; 32 : 1995-8.

- Chimi H, Rahmani M, Cillard J, Cillard P. Autooxydation des huiles d'olive : rôle des composés phénoliques. *Rev Fr Corps Gras* 1990 ; 37 : 363-7.

- Choi HS, Moore DD. Induction of c-fos and c-jun gene expression by phenolic antioxidants. *Mol Endocrinol* 1993 ; 7 : 1596-602.

- Connor WE, Connor SL. Dietary fatty acids and cholesterol : effects on the plasma lipids and lipoproteins. In : Woodford FP, Davignon J, Sniderman A, eds. *Atherosclerosis X*. Amsterdam : Elsevier Science, 1995 : 275-83.

- Esteva P, Baudet MF, Lasserre M, Jacotot B. Influence of the fatty acid composition of high density lipoprotein phospholipids on the cholesterol efflux from cultured fibroblasts. *Biochim Biophys Acta* 1986 ; 875 : 174-82.

- Fernandez MA, Saenz MT, Garcia MD. Anti-inflammatory activity in rats and mice of phenolic acids isolated from Scrophularia frutescens. *J Pharm Pharmacol* 1998 ; 50 : 1183-6.

- Forcadell MLI, Comas M, Miquel X, De La Torre MC. Détermination du tyrosol et de l'hydroxytyrosol dans les huiles vierges d'olive. *Rev Fr Corps Gras* 1987 ; 34 : 547-9.

- Garg A, Bonanome A, Grundy SM, Zhang ZJ, Unger RH. Comparison of a high carbohydrate diet with a high-monounsaturated – fat diet in patients with non-insulin-dependent diabetes melitus. *N Engl J Med* 1988 ; 319 : 829-34.

- Ginsberg HN, Barr SL, Gilbert A, Karmally W, Deckelbaum R, Kaplan K, Rama Krishnan R, Holleran S, Dell RB. Reduction of plasma cholesterol levels in normal men on an american heart association step 1 diet or a step 1 diet with added monounsaturated fats. *N Engl J Med* 1990 ; 322 : 574-9.

- Grundy SM. Comparison of monounsaturated fatty acids and carbohydrates for lowering plasma cholesterol. *N Engl J Med* 1986 ; 314 : 745-8.

- Haumann BF. Olive oil. *Inform* 1996 ; 7 : 890-903.

- Herbert JM, Maffrand JP, Taoubi K, Augereau JM, Fouraste I, Gleye J. Verbascoside isolated from Lantana camara, an inhibitor of protein kinase C. *J Nat Prod* 1991 ; 54 : 1595-600.

- Howell TJ, MacDougall DE, Jones PJH. Phytosterols partially explain differences in cholesterol metabolism caused by corn or olive oil feeding. *J Lipid Res* 1998 ; 39 : 892-900.

- Hu FB, Stampfer MJ, Manson JE, *et al*. Dietary fat intake and the risk of coronary heart disease in women. *N Engl J Med* 1997 ; 337 : 1491-9.

- Jornot L, Junod AF. Hyperoxia, unlike phorbol ester, induces glutathione peroxidase through a protein kinase C-independent mechanism. *Biochem J* 1997 ; 326 : 117-23.

- Keys A, Fidanga F, Scardi V, Bergami G, Keys MH, Lorenzo F. Studies on serum cholesterol and other characteristics of clinically healthy men in Naples. *Arch Intern Med* 1954 ; 93 : 328-36.

- Keys A. Diet and the epidemiology of coronary heart disease. *JAMA* 1957 ; 164 : 1912.

- Keys A, Menotti A, Karvonen MJ, Aravanis C, Blackbuen H, Buzina R, Djordjevic BS, Dontas AS, Fidanza F, Keys MH. The diet and 15-year death rate in the seven countries study. *Am J Epidemiol* 1986 ; 124(6) : 903-15.

- Köhrle J, Auf'mkolk M, Spanka M, Irmscher K, Cody V, Hesh RD. Iodothyronine deiodinaseis inhibited by plant flavonoids. In : Cody V, Middleton E Jr, Harborne JB, Beretz A, eds. *Plant flavonoids in biology and medicine : biochemical, pharmacological and structure-activity relationships*. New York : Alan R. Liss Inc, 1986 : 359-71.

- Kohyama N, Nagata T, Fujimoto S, Sekiya K. Inhibition of arachidonate lipoxygenase activities by 2-(3,4-dihydroxyphenyl)ethanol, a phenolic compound from olives. *Biosci Biotechnol Biochem* 1997 ; 61 : 347-50.

- Koshihara Y, Neichi T, Murota S, Lao A, Fujimato Y, Tatsuno T. Caffeic acid is a selective inhibitor for leukotriene biosynthesis. *Biochem Biophys Acta* 1984 ; 792 : 92-7.

- Kromhout D, Menotti A, Blackburn H, eds. *The seven countries study : a scientific adventure in cardiovascular disease epidemiology*. Utrecht (Netherlands) : Brouwer Offset, 1994.

- Laval-Jeantet AM. Évaluation du rôle protecteur de l'huile d'olive dans l'ostéoporose liée au vieillissement et à la ménopause. Rapport à la Communauté Économique Européenne, 1983.

- Laval-Jeantet AM, Gen P, Bergot C, Lamarque JL, N'Guiania M. Correlation between bone density measurement and nutritional status. In : Christiansen, ed. *Osteoporosis*. Copenhague, 1984 : 305-9.

- Lopez-Segura F, Velasco F, Lopez-Miranda J, *et al.* Monounsaturated fatty acid-enriched diet decreases plasma plasminogen activator inhibitor type 1. *Arterioscler Thromb Vasc Biol* 1996 ; 16 : 82-8.

- Luchetti F. Situation et perspectives du marché international de l'huile d'olive. *OCL* 1997 ; 4 : 336-7.

- Mattson FH, Grundy SM. Comparison of effects of dietary saturated, monounsaturated and polyunsaturated fatty acids on plasma lipids and lipoproteins in man. *J Lipid Res* 1985 ; 26 : 194-202.

- Mensink RP, de Groot MJ, van den Broeke LT, Severijnen-Nobels AP, Demacker PN, Katan MB. Effects of monounsaturated fatty acids *versus* complex carbohydrates on serum lipoproteins and apoproteins in healthy men and women. *Metabolism* 1989 ; 38 : 172-8.

- Mensink RP, Katan MB. Effect of monounsaturated fatty acids *versus* complex carbohydrates on high density lipoproteins in healthy men and women. *Lancet* 1987 ; 1 : 122-5.

- Mensink RP, Katan MB. Effect of a diet enriched with monounsaturated or polyunsaturated fatty acids on levels of low-density and high-density lipoprotein cholesterol in healthy women and men. *N Engl J Med* 1989 ; 321 : 436-41.

- Middleton Jr E, Ferriola P. Effect of flavonoids on protein kinase C : relationship to inhibition of human basophil histamine release. In : Cody V, Middleton E Jr, Harborne JB, Beretz A, eds. *Plant flavonoids in biology and medicine : biochemical, cellular and medicinal properties*. New York : Alan R. Liss Inc, 1988 : 251-66.

- Miettinen TA, Vanhanen H. Serum concentration and metabolism of cholesterol during rapeseed oil and squalene feeding. *Am J Clin Nutr* 1994 ; 59 : 356-63.

- Natarajan K, Singh S, Burke TR Jr, Grunberger D, Aggarwal BB. Caffeic acid phenethyl ester is a potent and specific inhibitor of activation of nuclear transcription factor NF-kappaB. *Proc Natl Acad Sci USA* 1996 ; 93 : 9090-5.

- Nydahl MC, Gustafsson IB, Vessby B. Lipid-lowering diets enriched with monounsaturated or polyunsaturated fatty acids but low in saturated fatty acids have similar effects on serum lipid concentrations in hyperlipidemic patients. *Am J Clin Nutr* 1994 ; 59 : 115-22.

- Parhami F, Morrow AD, Balucan J, Leitinger N, Watson AD, Tintut Y, Berliner JA, Demer LL. Lipid oxidation products have opposite effects on calcifying vascular cell and bone cell differentiation. A possible explanation for the paradox of arterial calcification in osteoporotic patients ? *Arterioscler Thromb Vasc Biol* 1997 ; 17 : 680-7.

- Parthasarathy S, Khoo JC, Miller E, Barnett J, Witztum JL, Steinberg D. Low density lipoprotein rich in oleic acid is protected against oxidative modification : implications for dietary prevention of atherosclerosis. *Proc Natl Acad Sci USA* 1990 ; 87 : 3894-8.

- Parthasarathy S, Rankin SM. Role of oxidized low density lipoprotein in atherogenesis. *Prog Lipid Res* 1992 ; 31 : 127-43.

- Perrin JL. Les composés mineurs et les antioxygènes naturels de l'olive et de son huile. Mise au point. *Rev Fr Corps Gras* 1992 ; 39 : 25-32.

- Petroni A, Blasevich M, Salami M, Papini N, Montedoro GF, Galli C. Inhibition of platelet aggregation and eicosanoid production by phenolic components of olive oil. *Thromb Res* 1995 ; 78 : 151-60.

- Scaccini C, Nardini M, D'Aquino M, Gentili V, Di Felice M, Tomassi G. Effect of dietary oils on lipid peroxidation and on antioxidant parameters of rat plasma and lipoprotein fractions. *J Lipid Res* 1992 ; 33 : 627-33.

- Selway JWT. Antiviral activity of flavones and flavans. In : Cody V, Middleton E Jr, Harborne JB, Beretz A, eds. *Plant flavonoids in biology and medicine : biochemical, pharmacological and and structure-activity relationships*. New York : Alan R. Liss Inc, 1986 : 521-36.

- Suzuki YJ, Packer L. Inhibition of NF-kB DNA binding activity by alpha-tocopherol succinate. *Biochem Mol Biol Int* 1993a ; 31 : 693-700.

- Suzuki YJ, Packer L. Inhibition of NF-kB DNA binding activity by catechol derivatives. *Biochem Mol Biol Int* 1993b ; 32 : 299-305.

- Tsimidou M, Papadopoulos G, Boskou D. Phenolic compounds and stability of virgin olive oil – Part 1. *Food Chem* 1992 ; 45 : 141-4.

• Uzzan A. *Manuel des corps gras, olive et huile d'olive*. 1992 : 221-8.

• Vazquez Roncero A. Les polyphénols de l'huile d'olive et leur influence sur les caractéristiques de l'huile. *Rev Fr Corps Gras* 1978 ; 25 : 21-6.

• Vicario IM, Malkova D, Lund EK, Johnson IT. Olive oil supplementation in healthy adults : effects in cell membrane fatty acid composition and platelet function. *Ann Nutr Metab* 1998 ; 42 : 160-9.

• Visioli F, Bellomo G, Montedoro GF, Galli C. Low density lipoprotein oxidation is inhibited *in vitro* by olive oil constituents. *Atherosclerosis* 1995 ; 117 : 25-32.

• Visioli F, Bellosta S, Galli C. Oleuropein, the bitter principle of olives, enhances nitric oxide production by mouse macrophages. *Life Sci* 1998 ; 62 : 541-6.

• Welton AF, Tobias LD, Fiedler-Nagy C, Anderson W, Hope W, Meyers K, Coffey JW. The effect of flavonoids on arachidonic acid metabolism. In : Cody V, Middleton E Jr, Harborne JB, Beretz A, eds. *Plant flavonoids in biology and medicine : Biochemical, pharmacological and structure-activity relationships*. New York : Alan R. Liss Inc, 1986 : 231-42.

• Wilson PW, Abbott RD, Castelli WP. High density lipoprotein cholesterol and mortality. The Framingham Heart Study. *Arteriosclerosis* 1988 ; 8 : 737-41.

• Wiseman SA, Mathot JNNJ, De Fouw NJ, Tijburg LBM. Dietary non-tocopherol antioxidants present in extra virgin olive oil increase the resistance of low density lipoproteins to oxidation in rabbits. *Atherosclerosis* 1996 ; 120 : 15-23.

• Wisout K. Lipids and Cancer. *Inform* 1999 ; 10(5) : 380-97.

• Wolk A, Bergstrom R, Hunter D, Wille HW, Ljung H, Holmberg L, Bergkvist L, Bruce A, Adami HO. A prospective study of association of mono unsaturated fat and other types of fat with risk of breast cancer. *Arch Intern Med* 1998 ; 158 : 41-5.

Fish and sea foods

Mariette Gerber, Luçay Han-Ching, Gérard Pieroni

The epidaemiological studies that generated the hypothesis, according to which the consumption of fish has a beneficial effect on health, were reported in the first chapter of this book. It has been seen that in general there are few of these studies, and analytical studies are particularly scarce. However, they strongly suggest a protective effect for cardiovascular diseases, while there are fewer data for cancer.

In the case of this food, as in most of the ones we study, the mechanisms have been better elucidated for cardiovascular diseases than for cancers. The reason, previously mentioned, is that there are intermediary markers in cardiovascular diseases; these markers are often absent in the natural history of cancers.

Fatty acids from fish oil

Fish oils contain long chain poly-unsaturated fatty acids with 20 or more carbon atoms (LC-PUFA). Humans cannot synthesise the amounts of LC-PUFA required for the proper functioning of their bodies. Therefore, LC-PUFA must be provided by diet. LC-PUFA are not found in terrestrial plants, they are essentially found in offal from mammals and in fish and sea foods that are a rich source. In the latter, it is mainly eicosapentanoic acid (EPA) with 20 carbon atoms and 5 double bonds and docosohaxaenoic (DHA) with 22 carbon atoms and 6 double bonds. They are said to belong to the n-3 series as the first double bond is on carbon 3.

Fish oils seem to have a beneficial effect on humoral lipid parameters and an anti-fibrillation effect on cardiac muscle, which agrees with the observation of Daviglus *et al.* (1997) of the maximum effect of the reduction on death risk in the days following a myocardial infarction.

For cancers based on animal studies, studies of mammary tumours in rats showed a slowing down in tumour growth accompanied by an increase in intra-tumour necrosis in animals supplemented with cold water fish oil (reviewed in Bougnoux *et al.*, 1996). The large proportion of polyunsaturated n-3 series fatty acids, eicosapentanoic (EPA) and docosohaxaenoic (DHA) decreased arachidonic acid synthesis, inducing a decrease of the products derived from its metabolism. The decrease in the synthesis of thromboxane results in haemorrhages, thus intra-tumour necrosis, and the decrease in prostaglandins reduces tumour progression and the appearance of metastases.

> **Arachidonic acid metabolic path**
>
> Arachidonic acid (C20:4 n-6) is a poly-unsaturated fatty acid (4 double bonds) with a long 20 carbon atom chain, belonging to the n-6 series (first double bond on carbon 6). This fatty acid is at the origin of two metabolic paths regulated by PGH synthetase (enzyme previously called cyclo-oxigenase) that synthesises the first form of prostaglandin (PG) precursor of other PGs, and the lipo-oxigenases family that involve the cyclo-oxigenase enzyme, respectively. The first catalyses the synthesis of special compounds, such as thromboxane, involved in coagulation phenomena and vessel constriction, and prostaglandins, involved in inflammatory reactions and cellular migration. The second specifically catalyses the synthesis of pro-inflammatory leukotrienes (LTB4). The n-3 series fatty acids decrease the synthesis of products derived from C20: 4 n-6.

However, both for cardiovascular diseases and for cancers, the fish-meat substitution effect cannot be eliminated, which allows the decrease of the impact of the risk factors related to meat consumption (*see chapter* "Health benefits of the Mediterranean eating model").

Therefore, it would seem that nutritional recommendations must integrate a replacement of land meat products by products of sea origin, and to a currently badly defined extent. The advice remains vague both in the food allowance "pyramid" (WHO, 1994, *see chapter* "Preserve and promote Mediterranean food for health"), and in the recommendations of the *American Heart Association* (Krauss *et al.*, 1996). In the Lyon study (de Lorgeril *et al.*, 1994), the "Mediterranean" type intervention did not include any more detail on fish consumption than the recommendations of the American Heart Association. In a study of primary prevention of the cardiovascular risk factors by the Mediterranean diet that we carry out in Marseilles (Philippe Vague and the CDPA, Denis Lairon and the INSERM Unit 476, Mariette Gerber and the Metabolic Epidemiology Group, Montpellier, Michel Rotily and ORS PACA), the consumption of fish is present in 5 of the 7 main meals in the week.

If we recommend the consumption of fish, the problems of distribution and supply may come up in the short term, in view of the difficulties in preservation and the deterioration of fish resources.

Breeding and fish-farming may provide an answer to these questions, however they bring the problem of the diet of the farmed fish that may lose their characteristics depending on the nutrients making up their diet.

The two contributions proposed provide answers to this problem, since one treats the problem of freezing, therefore the appropriate preservation of nutrients of interest in fish supplied to consumers, and the other the addition of the fatty acids EPA and DHA to other foods and eggs.

EFFECTS OF PRESERVATION ON FISH POLY-UNSATURATED FATTY ACIDS

The meat of fish is organised in layers and presents itself as two types of muscles: red muscle and white muscle. Its carbohydrate content is insignificant, it contains 18 to 20% proteins and 1 to 25% of lipids, depending whether we are considering lean fish, fatty fish or intermediate fish; however the variability is still large within the fatty fish class.

For this reason, the caloric value of fish varies between 80 kcal/100 g to 300 kcal/100 g.

Another difference to be introduced is that between caught fish, or so called "wild", and fish from farming, which have a less variable composition, as it essentially depends on the diet provided. The meat is generally fattier.

Lipid composition of fish meat

A lipid reserve is required by fish; it is made up of triglycerides and is located in the liver for lean fish and in muscle for fatty fish.

There are also transmembrane lipids that represent less than 1% of total lipids in fish; these are phospholipids (phosphatidyl choline and phosphatidyl ethanolamine). The fatty acids of these lipids contain a greater proportion of unsaturated fatty acids than the triglycerides that make up the lipid reserve.

The fatty acids found in fish are described in *Table I*.

Table I. Fatty acid composition of different fish expressed in g per 100 g of total fatty acids

	Cod[1] (cooked in the oven)	Sardine[2] (raw)	Herring[1] (grilled)	Horse mackerel[2] (raw)
Total fatty acids	1	9	12.3	9
Saturated fatty acids	26	31	23	29
Mono-unsaturated fatty acids	16	34	56	41
Poly-unsaturated fatty acids	58	33	20	27
• EPA (C20: 5 n-3)	17.5	16	7.2	8
• DHA (C22: 6 n-3)	35	8	6.7	11
Others	1.2	2	3	3

[1] Simopoulos (1997).
[2] source: IFREMER data (period: winter - zone: Brittany).

It can be seen that the fatty acid spectrum found in fish is wider than fatty acids of land origin. In particular, they contain more unsaturated fatty acids than land animals. Polyunsaturated fatty acids represent 20 to 60% of total fatty acids, especially EPA (C20: 5 n-3) and DHA (C22: 6 n-3), as there is on average a ratio of n-6/n-3? 0.16 for temperate water fish, and a higher ratio for warm water fish.

In practice, it may be stated that lean fish contain approximately 300 mg of n-3 fatty acids/100 g of meat, with a predominance of DHA and fatty fish 1 to 5 g of n-3 fatty acids/100 g of meat.

Therefore, it is essential to preserve these fatty acid characteristics of fish. We will present the conditions for this preservation, those related to the tissue make up of the fish meat and its evolution, and those related to the preservation treatments.

Preservation conditions related to the tissue characteristics of fish

Compounds naturally present in fish tissue can act as pro-oxidants and anti-oxidants.

Rapidly after death, a series of biochemical phenomena favouring lipid oxidation is observed.

Initiation of oxidation in fish meat

Initially there is a decrease in reducing compounds (NAD(P)H, glutathion and ascorbate), a release of metal compounds, activation of myoglobin and methaemoglobin by H_2O_2, an increase in Ca^{++} concentration resulting in enzymatic activation, the disintegration of cellular membranes, and a loss of fat soluble anti-oxidants.
This phase is followed by an auto-oxidation process of the lipids.

The importance of these post-mortem phenomena will partly condition the evolution of the conservation of fatty acids during preservation procedures. However, oxidation criteria are little used to evaluate the quality of fresh fish.

Preservation conditions related to the preservation techniques

Refrigeration

During refrigeration, lipid degradation manifests itself by a release of free fatty acids, the initiation of oxidation and the appearance of early oxidation products and sometimes even at this stage, an oxidation that can be observed on the ventral wall. The intensity of these alterations depends on the biological conditions described above and the handling conditions prior to refrigeration. When the handling conditions have not been controlled upstream, the results concerning the evolution of fatty acids, especially n-3, and their degradation level at the refrigerated state will be very variable.

In general, it can be said that tocopherol (vitamin E) rapidly decreases during the first days of storage, while an increase in conjugated dienes and trienes is progressively observed.

Freezing

Several factors favour oxidation in the frozen state:

– possible initiation prior to freezing, followed by not well controlled handling, especially the bleeding,
– effect of the salt concentration which have a catalyst role,
– lipases and phospholipases still active at $-30\,°C$,

– mechanical damage of cellular membranes,
– superficial tissue dehydration.

This would have practical consequences on the oxidation of lipids present in lean fish and fatty fish. This is the main factor limiting the duration of conservation of fatty fish, and the oxidation criteria are widely used to evaluate the quality of frozen fish. Oxidation may be worsened by bad storage conditions, but anyway, there is a tendency to a progressive and regular decrease of EPA and DHA during storage in frozen state.

Aseptic canning

With respect to aseptic canning, the main problem lies in the handling and storage conditions prior to aseptic canning. The following can exist:

– a chain proxidation in the refrigerated conditions and often in the frozen conditions prior to aseptic canning,

– high temperature conditions during the operations prior to sterilisation (thawing, trimming, packing).

Too high temperatures during aseptic canning will favour carbonyl-amine type chemical reactions between lipid oxidation products and free amine groups from proteins (Schiff's base).

However, during the storage of canned fish, EPA and DHA contents remain stable.

Comparison of EPA and DHA contents and evolution of frozen and canned products (Rougereau and Person, 1991)

In canned mackerels in vinegar, EPA and DHA content remains constant over a period of 2 years, while it decreases during storage in a frozen state over a period of one year. For canned sardines in oil, from the beginning a decrease in EPA and DHA content in the meat is observed due to the migration of the compounds into the covering oil. However, after equilibration the content remains the same during a storage period of 2 years. In the frozen state, the content of these fatty acids remains relatively stable at first and then tends to decrease.

Unfortunately, in the two cases of the frozen state study, neither the treatment conditions of the raw material nor the level of evolution of their lipids before freezing were specified. However, it remains that freezing does not provide a stability comparable to that of canning and for this reason, to maintain a sufficient quality of frozen products, the conservation expiry date must be adjusted according to the initial conditions of the raw material and the storage and packing conditions.

Conclusions

The following must be emphasised:

– the importance of the early steps: fishing conditions and storage on board,

– the difference of behaviour of (fatty) fish as a function of the sexual cycle,

- the little evolution of n-3 fatty acids in good practice conditions and control of freshness of raw material for all the conservation methods in general,
- the little effect of refrigeration on n-3 fatty acids in practice,
- the effect of the duration of storage in the frozen state which tends to result in a decrease in the concentration of n-3 fatty acids,
- the stability of n-3 fatty acids after aseptic canning.

MARINE LIPIDS AND HUMAN DIET

Fatty acids are molecules that are essential for life, and constitute the main portion of lipids from living beings. They fill essentially three major functions as participants in:
- cell structure,
- intracellular, intercellular and inter-organ communication,
- provision of energy to cells.

Long chain poly-unsaturated fatty acids (LC-PUFA) synthesised in small amounts from precursors, the essential fatty acids, which are relatively abundant in food participate in the building of cellular structures and communication functions.

In many situations humans are incapable of synthesising the amounts of LC-PUFA required for the proper function of their bodies. Therefore, LC-PUFA must be provided by food. LC-PUFA are not found in the terrestrial vegetable world, they are essentially found in the offal of mammals and in fish and sea foods that are a rich source.

The evolution in dietary habits has resulted in a reduction of the consumption of offal from mammals. The use of fish and sea-foods, in spite of the progress in the cold chain and the opportunities offered by freezing, run into the acquired habits which only include fish in a very marginal manner in the composition of meals. Furthermore, the LC-PUFA content of fish and sea-foods can vary to a large extent according to the nature of the product, its geographical origin, season, whether it is wild or farmed, how it has been cooked, and once on the plate, the portion consumed. Conservation in ice after catching, by deep-freezing as well as the treatments, filleting, canning, and cooking also greatly influence the maintenance of the integrity of the LC-PUFA *(see previous paragraph)*.

Little interest is granted to LC-PUFA content in food. This field remains to be explored. There is insufficient knowledge on the effects of LC-PUFA on health obtained from large epidemiological studies. The question is all the more important as sea LC-PUFA do not have all the same effects on human health and they are found in variable proportions depending on the product concerned.

Industrial fish oils obtained from well defined species have much more reduced variations in LC-PUFA composition, often limited to seasonal variations due to the mass treated and the possibilities of mixing. Therefore, they present themselves as well defined starting materials that begin to be proposed now as ingredients for the food industry. It should be reminded that hydrogenated fish oil has been used in human food since the beginning of the XIXth century and that after hydrogenation there are no LC-PUFA left. Non hydrogenated oils have a reputation of being very sensitive to oxidation and must be protected from oxygen in air, light and high temperatures. Technological advances have resulted in a micro-encapsulated form, which looks like a flour. Micro-encapsulation improves oxidation resistance.

Fat hydrogenation

Transformation technique employed on unsaturated lipids and oils, and consists in the saturation of double bonds by binding hydrogen. Due to this the oils become solids: the decrease in the number of double bonds and the modification of those that resist (trans situation) result in an alteration of the physico-chemical properties making them behave like saturated fats. The same applies with respect to the relation of saturated fats to degenerative chronic diseases, as they appear as risk factors.

Another approach consists in using these oils as animal feed supplements. This use is not new; what is new is the follow-up of the LC-PUFA composition carried out in the animal products obtained, as well as the incidence on human health which ensues from the consumption of such products. A European project, entitled Eureka and involving Spain and Holland, has been launched concerning the enrichment of chicken meat, as well as eggs and pork meat with LC-PUFA. Projects concerning the enrichment of bovine meat, as well as milk, are also in progress.

Our experience involves in particular hen eggs where the poly-unsaturated fatty acid, and thus LC-PUFA composition can be easily modified by diet. The addition of fish oil to poultry feed allows the enrichment of egg lipids in LC-PUFA and this can be done with some specificity with respect to the different LC-PUFA. This results in eggs that can present in a way lipid compositions on demand. Thus, eggs appear as a form of fish LC-PUFA controlled supplement for humans. Eggs, egg-products and derivatives containing these LC-PUFA are likely to have different properties for human health. The demonstration of these effects results in work that is being developed. It can be envisaged, if interesting results are observed, to purify the active ingredients in order to obtain nutritional supplements. It would be a fine Odyssey for an oil that is initially a sub-product of fish meals, sub-products of industrial fishing.

CONCLUSION

It would seem beneficial for human health to increase the proportion in fish and sea-food intake in the diet. A greater spread of this product must be accompanied by a reflection on its availability and distribution.

The importance of the treatment of fish before reaching the consumer and before the conservation methods has been examined. The consumer, the "preservers" and the "transformer" must be informed of the quality of the treatments and the objective criteria of this quality could be used by the "preservers" and the "transformers". The good behaviour of some canned products, too often neglected, must be emphasised.

The improvement in the "preservation" and "transformation" fields will perhaps not be sufficient to guarantee a distribution of fish and sea-foods likely to influence Public Health. The use of the addition of beneficial fatty acids to other foods may be an interesting track, even if it seems inappropriate to the partisans of traditional Mediterranean diet.

REFERENCES

- Bandarra NM, Undeland I, Nunes ML, Batista I, Empis JM. Lipid oxydation indices to evaluate sardine freshness. In : *Evaluation of fish freshness – AIR CT 942283*. Nantes, France : Institut International du Froid, 1997 : 263-5.

- Bougnoux P, Corpet D, Gerber M. Acides gras alimentaires et cancerogenèse. *Alimentation et cancer*. Paris : Lavoisier Tec Doc, 1996.

- Daviglus ML, Stamler J, Orencia AJ, Dyer AR, Liu K, Greenland P, Walsh MK, Morris D, Shekelle RB. Fish consumption and the 30-year risk of fatal myocardial infarction. *N Engl J Med* 1997 ; 336 : 1046-53.

- De Lorgeril M, Renaud S, Mamelle N, *et al*. Mediterranean alpha-linolenic acid rich diet in secondary pevention of coronary heart disease. *Lancet* 1994 ; 343 : 1454-9.

- Krauss RM, Deckelbaum RJ, Ernst N, Fisher E, Howard BV, Knopp RH, Kotchen T, Lichtenstein AH, McGill HC, Perseon TA, Prewitt TE, Stone NJ, Horn LV, Weinberg R. Dietary guidelines for healthy american adults. A statement for health professionals from the Nutrition Committee, American Heart Association. *Circulation* 1996 ; 94 : 1795-800.

- OMS Europe. Oldways preservation & exchange trust, WHO/FAO collaborating Center for Nutriton at Harvard Scool of Public Health, 1994.

- Rougereau A, Person O. Intérêt nutritionnel des acides gras insaturés de la sardine et du maquereau – Influence du mode de conservation. *Med Nutr* 1991 ; XXVII, 6 : 353-8.

- Simopoulos AP. Nutritional aspects of fish. In : Luten JB, Borresen T, Oehlenschlager J, eds. *Seafoods from producer to consumer. Integrated approach to quality*. Amsterdam : 1997 ; 589-607.

Wine consumption and cardiovascular disease prevention

Claude-Louis Léger, Marie-Annette Carbonneau, Bernard Descomps

EPIDEMIOLOGICAL STUDIES – BRIEF REMINDER

The epidemiological studies analysing the relationship between alcohol or alcoholic beverage consumption and cardiovascular disease in humans have been recently reviewed (Carando *et al.*, 1998a; Carando *et al.*, 1998b; see also the chapter "Health benefits of the Mediterranean consumption model"). They generally conclude that moderate alcoholic beverage drinkers have a reduced risk of cardiovascular diseases (CVD), in comparison with abstinent subjects or excessive drinkers. The situation is more ambiguous in terms of the specific advantages relative to each type of alcoholic beverage. Out of four cohort studies reported (Carando *et al.*, 1998b), one concludes to the absence of effect of wine consumption. For the three others, two show an effect of wine equal to that of beer or spirits, and one gives an advantage to wine in terms of total mortality (*see chapter* "Health benefits of the Mediterranean consumption model"). In a recent study on 40,000 individuals, mainly wine drinkers, from the Nancy region, the consumption of 2 to 3 wine glasses per day (21 to 32 g of alcohol/day) significantly decreases, on average by 35%, the risk of cardiovascular mortality (Renaud *et al.*, 1998), but the dietary habits (apart from drinks) of the subjects are not taken into account, which, as will be seen in other chapters, are involved on the level of cardiovascular risk. Finally, the data in press from the MONICA-France study are reported in the chapter "Health benefits of the Mediterranean consumption model". Thus when the risk of cardiovascular disease or the reliable indicators of risk are examined, current data suggest that the different forms of alcohol intake are not equivalent, and that moderate wine drinking is not related to cardiovascular risk indicators or factors, or even to the usual indicators of alcohol drinking (android obesity, gamma-glutamyl-transferase (GGT)).

WINE CONSUMPTION AND DECREASE OF CARDIOVASCULAR DISEASE RISK: CAUSE EFFECT RELATIONSHIP?

Is there a causal relationship between moderate wine consumption and decrease in the cardiovascular risk that would make plausible the results of epidemiological studies? In other words, does at least one mechanism of action explain the beneficial effects that could be specifically attributed to wine by these studies?

The oxidative theory of atherosclerosis, definitively formulated in the beginning of the 1990s and based on a large number of converging results, provides investigators at present and in the future with clues of great interest in this research of causal relationship. The antioxidant protection mechanisms of biological or chemical structures are undoubtedly involved in cardiovascular protection, and especially in the protection due to wine. However, other mechanisms may also explain the beneficial effects of wine. We will briefly examine all these mechanisms, as well as the conditions for their existence. On the other hand, we will not discuss here the effect specifically related to alcohol for two reasons: its favourable effects on HDL-related cholesterolemia *(see glossary)* involve mechanisms totally dissociated from those we will mention here *(see chapter* "Health benefits of the Mediterranean consumption model"), and it does not seem to modify (and in particular improve) the bioavailability of antioxidant substances contained in wine *(see below)*.

ATHEROSCLEROSIS OXIDATIVE THEORY: OXIDIZED LDL, OXIDIZABILITY OF LDL AND ANTIOXIDANT CAPACITY OF PLASMA

According to the atherosclerosis oxidative theory, oxidized LDL (oxLDL) play a major role in the atherosclerotic process and several mechanisms it involves *(figure 1)* in the vascular wall.

The role attributed to oxLDL in atherosclerosis is not in contradiction with the predictive value of increased cholesterolemia, as a main risk factor in this pathology. On the contrary this role supplies:

– an explanation to the paradoxical status of certain populations (including the French population) who, in spite of presenting a high cholesterolemia and dietary lipid consumption relative to others, still have a lower cardiovascular mortality ratio; a decrease in oxLDL production by an increased natural protection of LDL due to dietary antioxidants may reconcile these data;
– an explanation of how the increase in LDL cholesterol (or LDL), may lead to the conditions for the initiation of oxLDL production by increasing the amounts of LDL present in contact and within the vascular wall, the preferential site of its oxidation.

It is also possible that antioxidants prevent the direct consequences of hypercholesterolemia since high cholesterol level has been found to be capable of decreasing natural protection of the vascular wall against a powerful oxidation agent (Ma *et al.*, 1997).

OxLDL do not seem to exist – or only exist in minute quantities – in blood circulation (Steinbrecher *et al.*, 1990, Ylä-Herttuala, 1998). They are only present in the vascular wall, in the

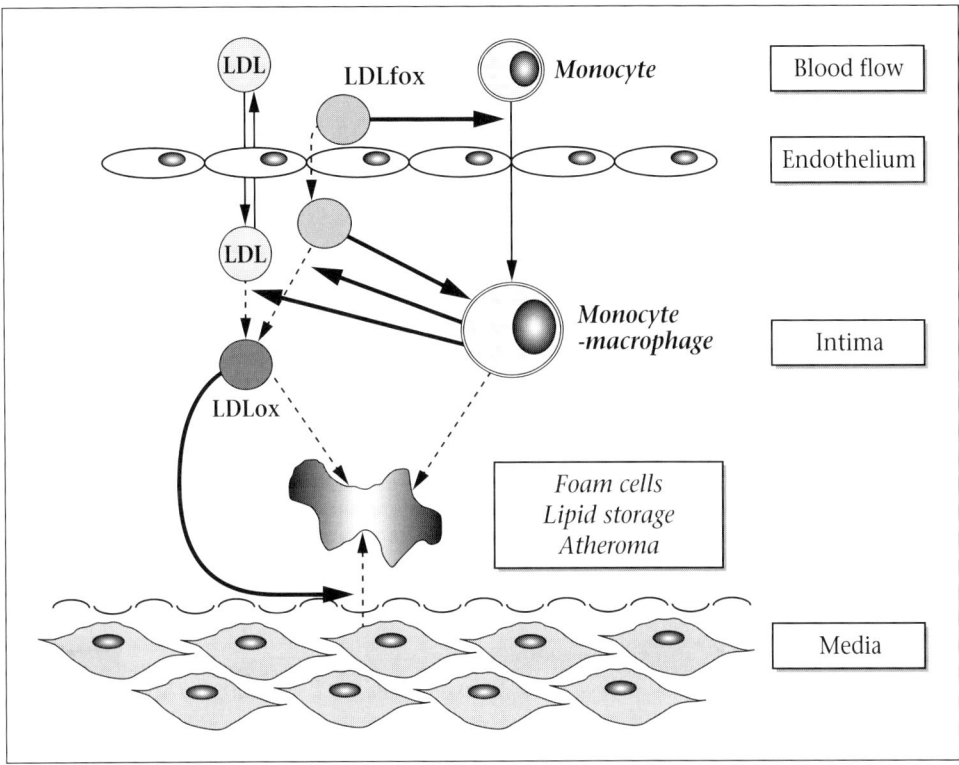

Figure 1. Atherogenic process in the vessel wall. Schematic section of the vessel wall with its three parts: endothelium in contact with the blood flow, the media made up of smooth muscle cells and the intima (or sub-endothelial space) which maintains the endothelial cells and muscular cells apart from each other. LDL in contact with the endothelium can undergo a transformation into minimally oxLDL. These will facilitate the passage of monocytes from the blood flow to the intima. Monocytes will in turn be activated by (minimally) oxLDL, which will result in an increased production of free radicals and will thus accentuate LDL oxidation. The increased production of oxLDL will lead to cells loaded with lipids called foam cells (which can also be produced by smooth muscle cells). Foam cells are among the basic cellular elements of the atheroma. The bold arrows represent the different types of action, the dashed arrows the transformations or movements of LDL or cells.

atheromatous lesion. However, the presence of oxLDL in plasma can be indirectly detected by assessing the plasma level of anti-oxLDL antibodies. This measurement shows that most longitudinal epidemiological studies support a statistical association between anti-oxLDL antibodies and increased cardiovascular risk, or in some cases between anti-oxLDL antibodies and increased severity of atherosclerotic attack (Salonen *et al.*, 1992; Puurunen *et al.*, 1994; Wu *et al.*, 1997).

Several processes *(Table I)* can lead to the oxidation of LDL *in vivo*.

Table I. Processes leading to LDL oxidation *in vivo*

Production of $O_2^{\cdot-}/HO\bullet_2^{\cdot}$ (with or without transition metals) by phagocytes (white blood cells capable of phagocytosis)	Bedwell *et al.* (1989)
Production of ClO$^-$ by myeloperoxidase of phagocytes or some polynuclear white blood cells	Savenkova *et al.* (1994) Daugherty *et al.* (1994)
By ONOO$^-$ produced by the reaction of $O_2^{\cdot-}$ with $^{\bullet}$NO from the endothelial cells (vessel cells in contact with blood)	Darley-Usmar *et al.* (1992) Wever *et al.* (1998)
Activity of 15-lipoxygenase	Kuhn *et al.* (1997)

$O_2^{\cdot-}/HO_2^{\cdot}$, ClO$^-$, ONOO$^-$, $^{\bullet}$NO are the superoxide ion and its conjugated acid, hypochlorous ion, peroxinitrite ion and nitrogen monoxide, respectively; these are all oxygen reactive species, but only the first and the last are radical species. They possess oxidant properties.

For simple practical reasons, the *ex vivo* measurement *(see glossary)* of the oxidation susceptibility (or oxidizability) of LDL and the opposite, the oxidation resistance, is often preferred to the detection of anti-oxLDL antibodies. It can be stated that the most oxidizable LDL are more likely to lead to oxLDL in the vascular wall resulting in a relationship between oxidizability and cardiovascular risk. This relationship has been demonstrated in a Northern European population (Regnström *et al.*, 1992), then confirmed in a Southern population (Cominacini *et al.*, 1993) and in an Asian population (Chin *et al.*, 1994).

In vitro oxidation of LDL

The problem posed by the LDL oxidation model commonly used for oxidizability determination should be emphasized. This model involves free copper, Cu^{2+}, which does not exist as such in the circulation and in the vascular wall. Therefore this poses the problem of the pathophysiological significance of this measurement. There are other systems capable of oxidizing LDL *in vitro* (Table *II)* closer to physiological or pathophysiological conditions that should be used simultaneously in the future to have a more reliable and consistent evaluation of the antioxidant properties of polyphenols. This illustrates the general but specific problem of the choice of the best marker(s) of LDL oxidizability, itself considered as an indicator of a pathological situation.

Table II. *In vitro* LDL oxidation systems

Type of system	Type of action involved
Cu^{2+} in the presence of O_2	Strictly chemical
Peroxide radical generators (ROO$^\bullet$)	Strictly chemical
Generators of the peroxinitrite ion (ONOO$^-$) or $O_2^\bullet$ + $^\bullet$NO (leading to ONOO$^-$)	Strictly chemical
$O_2^\bullet$ generator	Enzymatic or cellular
15-lipoxygenase (direct formation of fatty acid peroxides)	Enzymatic
Myeloperoxidase (production of ClO$^-$)	Enzymatic
Co-incubation of LDL + phagocytes	Cellular

As plasma is the medium in which LDL evolve naturally in the body, the measurement of the capacity of plasma to prevent oxidation leads to the evaluation of the *in vivo* LDL protection against oxidation by plasma. The measurement of plasma anti-oxidant capacity (PAOC) is easy *(see box below)*, however the value measured is characterized by an intra-individual variability that makes inter-individual comparisons difficult. Case-control studies are rare (Woodford and Whitehead, 1998). The usefulness of PAOC value as an indicator of cardiovascular risk has not been demonstrated up to now.

PAOC measurement

A plasma sample, usually less than 0.1 ml, is placed in a cuvette in the presence of a free radical generating system and luminol, a chemical substance that produces luminescence (emits light) when the capacity of the medium to scavenge free radicals is surpassed. The time elapsed until the appearance of luminescence (more precisely maximum half-luminescence) is measured. The longer the time, the greater the capacity of the plasma tested to protect itself from oxidation and to protect the chemical structures present in it (for example lipoproteins). For simplification purposes, this time is compared to that obtained with increasing concentrations of Trolox (a water soluble alpha-tocopherol analogue, alpha-tocopherol being one of the most common chemical forms of vitamin E). For this reason PAOC is frequently expressed in equivalent-Trolox/litre (EqT/l). Average values vary greatly from one population to another (from 0.2 to more than 1.0 mEqT/l)

PROTECTION AGAINST CARDIOVASCULAR DISEASES BY POLYPHENOLS – POSITION OF THE PROBLEM

In their different forms (flavanols, flavonols, phenolic acids and esterified derivatives), wine polyphenols (Cabanis *et al.*, 1998) are excellent antioxidants and, more specifically, excellent free radical scavengers *(see below)*. Therefore, if they are able to resist the physico-chemical conditions found within the stomach and the intestines, and the attacks of intestinal flora, they can pass through the intestinal wall into the blood and protect LDL from oxidation. They could thus have a protective role with respect to cardiovascular diseases. If the antioxidant wine-polyphenol properties *in vitro* towards LDL and *ex vivo* towards plasma are largely admitted, we are going to see that the results obtained after ingestion of wine polyphenols in healthy volunteers are rather inconsistent regarding their *in vivo* antioxidant protection of LDL, which results in real problems of interpretation.

Therefore, the questions currently asked to investigators could be summarised as follows: do polyphenols pass into the blood? Does the absorption of wine increase the plasma antioxidant capacity (PAOC) and/or the LDL oxidation resistance? Can other beneficial modifications related to wine consumption take place, especially in the vascular wall, to prevent atheroma and atherosclerosis?

PROTECTION OF LDL AGAINST OXIDATION *IN VITRO*

Studying *in vitro* antioxidant protection of LDL by polyphenols allows us to rank the different chemical species of polyphenols as a function of their antioxidant potency *(figure 2)*. Such a classification has to be related to the type of system used for generating oxidation. As these studies are commonly carried out with the system using Cu^{2+} and molecular oxygen *(see first line in Table II)*, the results obtained supply limited information. However, they have shown that catechin, epicatechin, procyanidins *(see technical information* "Polyphenols") dimers (B2, B3, B4), flavonols (rutin, myricetin, quercetin) and phenolic acids (caffeic acid, gallic acid) are among the most antioxidant polyphenols, by measuring the production of a fatty acid oxidation product (hexanal aldehyde) (Teissedre *et al.*, 1996; Frankel *et al.*, 1995). These results have been confirmed by the measurement of lag time of the conjugated diene (CD) production, which is the first manifestation (and an excellent indicator) of LDL oxidation *(figure 1 in the chapter* "Olive oil, olive oil by-products and olive fruit"). The polyphenols cited have in common an ortho-diphenol structure. It is interesting to note that the antioxidant capacity of polyphenols towards LDL depends on the presence of vitamin E in the LDL particle (Viana *et al.*, 1996). In the absence of vitamin E, polyphenols do not protect LDL against oxidation. This is important, as it suggests that *in vivo* the vitamin E content of LDL could partly control the protective capacity of polyphenols.

By comparing the Cu^{2+}/O_2 mediated oxidation of LDL to another oxidation generation system, it was possible to demonstrate that wine polyphenols acted partly as Cu^{2+} chelators, and that caffeic acid was one of the most protective phenolic compounds in the non Cu^{2+}-dependent system(Abu-Amsha *et al.*, 1996). These results illustrate the interest for investigators of a "diversification » of oxidation generating systems *(Table II)*.

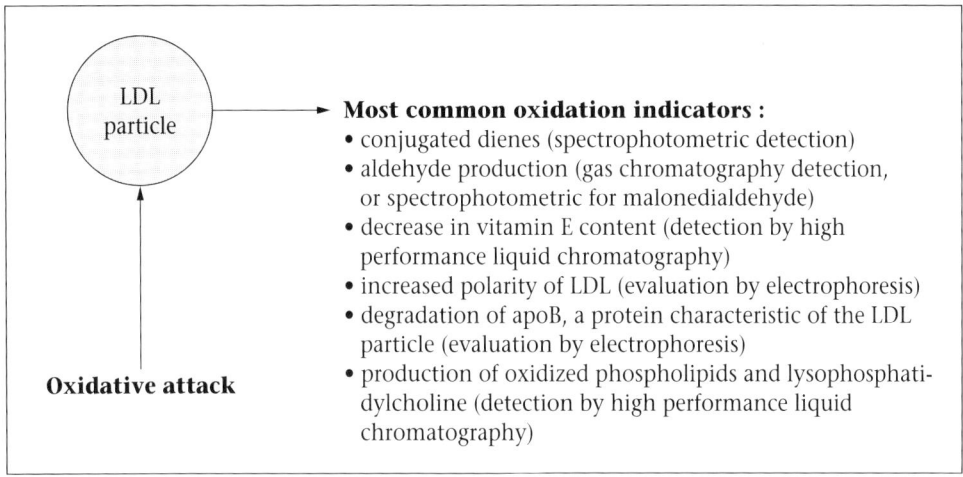

Figure 2. LDL oxidation indicators.

Different polyphenols are capable of scavenging radicals such as superoxide anion, peroxyl (Afanas'ev *et al.*, 1998; Torel *et al.*, 1987) and hydroxyl (Husain *et al.*, 1987). The important role of superoxide in the *in vivo* LDL oxidation was recently emphasized by investigators who used genomic over-expression of superoxide dismutase in aortic endothelial cells, a superoxide-degrading enzyme (Fang *et al.*, 1998). The protective role of polyphenols with respect to superoxide radicals is thus reinforced, as well as the ensuing pathological and physiological implications. Rutin chelates ferrous ion (Afanaz'ev *et al.*, 1998). Thus it can prevent the production of hydroxyl radical (the most reactive radical, as well as the most unstable due to its own reactivity) *via* Fenton reactions and play an antioxidant role. Catechin and epi-catechin (free or their gallo-derivatives) prevent the formation of nitro-tyrosine from peroxynitrite at concentrations below 10 µM and therefore, the formation of more polar modified LDL (Pannala *et al.*, 1997) capable of playing an atherogenic role.

THE ANTIOXIDANT EFFECT OF POLYPHENOLS *IN VIVO*

The first condition required for polyphenols to have an *in vivo* action that the investigator can demonstrate *ex vivo* or *in vivo* is that the constitutive molecule(s) pass the barrier of the intestinal wall, an essential condition for them to be present in the blood and intercellular medium.

Bioavailability of polyphenols

Intestinal absorption of conjugated or not conjugated flavonols (ex: quercetin, Hollman *et al.*, 1995), flavanols (ex: catechin, Hackett *et al.*, 1983) and phenolic acids (Woll *et al.*, 1995, and unpublished personal data) has been proven in humans today. However, major differences exist between these products, which have to be taken into account in order to get insight into their degree of "remanence" in blood (inverse of disappearance rate) and thus better determine their accumulation potential in the systemic medium.

After ingestion of food-supplied quercetin, the peak of quercetin is between 3 to 4 hours in plasma (Manach et al., 1998). When wine is drunk with a meal, preliminary results (unpublished personal data) indicate that the peak of catechin appears after the same time in plasma. Intestinal absorption of a flavanol (catechin) and a flavonol (quercetin) seems therefore to present comparable kinetic characteristics. When red wine is administered in fasting condition, Donovan et al. (1999) showed that the catechin and its derivatives peaked 1 hour after ingestion. Caffeic acid peaked within the first hour following the ingestion of red wine with a meal in the plasma (unpublished personal data), *i.e.* earlier than catechin under identical intake conditions. These results underscore the influence of the mode of wine consumption and of the chemical structure on absorption kinetics of polyphenols.

Maximum plasma levels of phenolic compounds after ingestion of red wine are strikingly different from one investigator group to another *(see box below)*.

Plasma phenolic compound levels after ingestion of red wine

The differences between results can be largely explained by the nature of the compound(s) analysed, and correlatively, by the analytical methods used. When the measurement carried out is based on plasma total polyphenol levels evaluated by the Folin-Ciocalteau reagent in fasting volunteers who had not taken any wine during the 2 weeks prior to the blood collection, Nigdikar et al. (1998) found concentrations of 16.2 mg/g of plasma protein, which corresponds to a plasma concentration of approximately 0.5 g/l for a minimally-estimated proteinemia of 30 g/l. This plasma concentration is greatly overestimated and seems not be compatible with the survival of the volunteers. After 2 weeks of a red wine intake of 375 ml/d, equivalent to 248 mg/d of polyphenols and including 70% as procyanidin polymers (number of monomers equal to or greater than 3), the concentration was found to increase from approximately 0.2 g/l to 0.7 g/l. In another study on fasting volunteers receiving 430 mg of total polyphenols as alcohol-free red wine (equivalent to 300 ml of alcohol-free red wine), Serafini et al. (1998) found that the plasma levels of polyphenols evaluated by the same reagent as above was between 7 mg/l (baseline value before ingestion) and 10 mg/l at the absorption plasma peak situated between 30 minutes and 2 hours after ingestion. The discrepancy between these two series of results can only be explained by methodological issues. Occurrence of plasma protein interference due to the use of the Folin-Ciocalteau in the first publication was minimized in the second as proteins were first precipitated.

These contradictory results reinforce the interest of separate measurements of the contents of each chemically identifiable phenolic wine constituent in the blood, a technically difficult task, but the only capable of providing accurate data on bioavailability. Such data are currently very few, but they are rather in accordance *(Table III)*. Plasma levels at the absorption peak following wine intake are close to 1 µg/l/mg of flavonoid ingested, and can fall to 0.5 µg/l/mg ingested in the case of a pharmacological dose administration (Hackett et al., 1983).

Table III. Level of identified polyphenols at the plasma absorption peak

Compound	Ingested amount (mg)	Plasma levels (mg/l)	References
Quercetin	90 (with meals)	0.12*	Manach et al. (1998)
Catechin	34 (fasting)	0.03*,#	Donovan et al. (1999)
Catechin	30 (with meals)	0.03	Unpublished personal data
Purified catechin	2000 (fasting)	1.0	Hackett et al. (1983)

* In equivalent quercetin or catechin, to take into account all the plasma forms of quercetin or catechin (conjugated, methylated or sulphated) present.
# Alcohol ingestion, simultaneous or not, does not have an effect on plasma levels.

The bioavailability of molecules estimated under these intake conditions does not give any direct indication on the transepithelial intestinal flow *in vivo*. The degradation of these different flavonoids in intestinal lumen and in the systemic medium, as well as urinary excretion (approximately 50% of ingested catechin, according to Hackett *et al.*, 1983) is not taken into account. From this point of view, the production of phenolic acids by the intestinal flora resulting from the scission of the flavonoid heterocycle (Hollman, 1997) leads to underestimate the flavanols/flavonols transepithelial flow and overestimate that of phenolic acids, already present in wine. Finally, it is known that catechin administration in fasting condition leads to a remarkably high proportion of plasma catechin in the derivative form (Donovan *et al.*, 1999) (methylated, glucuronides, sulphated) especially of hepatic origin. Further research is required to verify if the plasma proportion of native catechin/catechin derivatives is affected by the intake mode (fasting or with a meal) of the catechin.

In fasting condition, residual catechin plasma levels prior to the intake of any polyphenol rich substance are low; less than 2 µg/l in 18 healthy volunteers (lower than the electrochemical detection threshold; work in progress in our laboratory), less than 0.6 µg/l expressed as catechin equivalent (to take into account all the catechin forms present) in 9 healthy volunteers (less than the mass spectrometry detection threshold after trimethylsilylation; Donovan *et al.*, 1999). For gallic acid and caffeic acid, our data indicate that the plasma levels are also lower than the electrochemical detection threshold (2 µg/l).

Effect on plasma oxido-protection

All current studies agree on the fact that red wine consumption increases PAOC (*see box* "Measurement of PAOC"), but not white wine consumption *(table IV)*. It has been found to increase, first, at the intestinal absorption peak after a single intake of wine, and second, after regular wine intake over several days in fasting condition. PAOC evolution was followed up over 24 h following ingestion of red wine with a meal and compared to that obtained without wine ingestion (submitted for publication). The peak value of the differential with or without wine is situated about 4 h after ingestion. Therefore, there seems to be a coincidence in the time between the catechin peak *(see above)* and the PAOC peak. Is there a cause-effect relationship between these data? It is an unresolved question today. In view of the previously mentioned results, catechin or quercetin total plasma levels do not seem to be compatible with an increase of the plasma antioxidant protection levels observed, if one considers the concentrations required *in vitro* to obtain this protection. Furthermore, it seems that the polymeric forms of catechin (procyanidins) which represent the most abundant part of flavanols in wine can only have a local action on the intestinal mucosa, as their high molecular mass is incompatible with a passage through the intestinal wall. Phenolic acids present in wine or newly formed in the body after wine ingestion could be involved in the increased PAOC.

Table IV. Increase in the anti-oxidant capacity of serum or plasma after ingestion of wine

Wine	Number of administrations Number of subjects	Quantity	Effect: hours after intake and variation[a]	Method	Reference
Red	1 10 subjects	384 ml	1-1.5 h +15%	Lag time	Maxwell et al., 1994
Red	1 9 subjects	300 ml	1 h +18%	Lag time	Whitehead et al., 1995
White	1 3 subjects	300 ml	2 h NS	Lag time	Whitehead et al., 1995
Red	2/day 8 subjects	400 ml/day for 15 days	12 h +20%	TBARS	Fuhrman et al., 1995
White	2/day 8 subjects	400 ml/day for 15 days	12 h negative	TBARS	Fuhrman et al., 1995
Red (PP*)	2/day 10 subjects	equivalent to 1 l/day for 14 days	12 h +9%	Lag time	Carbonneau et al., 1997
Red (alcohol-free)	1 8 elderly subjects	300 ml	0-4 h approx. +10%	3 methods	Cao et al., 1998
Red (alcohol-free)	1 10 subjects	equivalent to 300 ml of wine	50 min 14%	Lag time	Serafini et al., 1998
White (alcohol-free)	1 10 subjects	equivalent to 300 ml of wine	50 min 0%	Lag time	Serafini et al., 1998
Red	1 3 subjects	100 ml fasting	30 min ++	Fe^{3+} reduction	Duthie et al., 1998
Red	1 3 subjects	300 ml	3-4 min +40%	Lag time	Léger et al., unpublished

[a] For a single administration, the delay of appearance of the maximum value and the maximum variation are indicated;
* Total polyphenol extract administered in capsules.

Effect on LDL antioxidant protection

Results concerning the effect of wine intake are not in accordance on the oxidation resistance of LDL under *ex vivo* measurement conditions (Nigdikar *et al.* 1998; Fuhrman *et al.*, 1995; Carbonneau *et al.*, 1997). This is probably explained by the existence of many methodological variants in the preparation of LDL. The centrifugation method (this technical aspect will not be developed here) and the dialysis step (indispensable for the use of LDL after centrifugation) are among them. For example, it has been demonstrated that dialysis leads to the loss of LDL polyphenols (Cao *et al.*, 1998, Carbonneau *et al*, 1997). Other mild procedures allow the disassociation of LDL polyphenols (Carbonnneau *et al.*, 1998). Therefore, these results indicate that the most likely localisation of polyphenols is on the surface of the LDL, a localisation which is the most stable thermodynamically (it should be reminded that these substances have amphipathic characteristics) and which also allows a fast movement from the LDL on which they are "adsorbed" towards the surrounding liquid environment.

If LDL antioxidant protection after dialysis, *i.e.* after the loss of polyphenols, is not modified by the ingestion of polyphenols found in wine, this does not actually mean that LDL are not protected *in vivo*. It has been shown that LDL are significantly enriched in vitamin E after a regular intake of wine polyphenols for 14 days. Therefore, vitamin E, the main LDL antioxidant, seems to be protected and spared by the increase in PAOC due to the oral administration of polyphenols (Carbonneau *et al.*, 1997). This supports an antioxidant protection of LDL *in vivo*.

Finally, beyond the existing disagreements, most groups of researchers show – in a direct or indirect manner – that the antioxidant LDL protection increases after a prolonged wine (or wine polyphenols) intake. According to the oxidative theory of atherosclerosis, this is in favor of a prevention of atherogenic processes.

OTHER EFFECTS DUE TO WINE OR WINE POLYPHENOLS (*IN VITRO* OR *IN VIVO*)

The aortic wall of rats is directly sensitive *in vitro* to high doses of red wine polyphenolic extracts, which turn out to favour the relaxation of the vessels. The mechanism takes place via cellular action as the synthesis of nitric oxide (a vasorelaxant) increases (Andriambeloson *et al.*, 1997). One crucial question raised by this result is that it is unknown whether lower concentrations are really active in blood, and if the compounds known to be active *in vitro* are actually present *in vivo*.

Platelet aggregation intervenes in the thrombo-atherogenic process and aggravates the atheroma leading to an "advanced" atherosclerotic lesion. It also intervenes in thrombosis and acute cardiovascular disease resulting in premature and sudden death. Anti-aggregation effects have been attributed to wine. However, the substances responsible are not well established. Alcohol was pointed out in a study in humans (Pellegrini *et al.*, 1996), whereas polyphenols (tannins) was pointed out in a study in rats (Ruf *et al.*, 1995).

Inflammatory processes are highly involved in atherogenesis. The inhibitory action of flavonols on 5-lipoxygenase (which controls the pathway leading to the synthesis of LTB4, a pro-inflammatory leukotriene) and on cyclo-oxygenase (Moroney *et al.*, 1998) (leading to the synthesis of prostaglandins, some of which are vasoconstrictive and pro-aggregating) is often cited as supporting the decrease in the risk of cardiovascular disease, and as able to protect from inflammatory manifestations. According to the current information, the concentrations required for an anti-inflammatory action seem incompatible with the low concentrations that may be found in plasma after wine ingestion. Furthermore, the flavonols mentioned are generally quantitatively low, or even at trace levels in wine (Cabanis *et al.*, 1998). With respect to phenolic acids found in wine, anti-inflammatory properties have been observed in rats and mice, but it was stressed that their topical action was more marked than after oral administration (Fernandez *et al.*, 1998). The same is true for the protective effects against oxidative attack of lymphocyte DNA obtained with flavonols (mainly quercetin and its different glycosylated derivatives (Noroozi *et al.*, 1998)).

Surprisingly, procyanidin oligomers prevented oxidative stress (Tebib *et al.*, 1997) and hypercholesterolemia in rats (Tebib *et al.*, 1994). An oxidative-stress prevention is defined here as an action that opposes the pro-oxidant effect of a prolonged vitamin E deficiency (therefore, opposing the decrease in tissue glutathion and increase in malondialdehyde), and that increases the expression of enzymes whose the function is to destroy the reactive oxygen species (ROS) in the body (the superoxide dismutase/glutathion peroxydase system, catalase). Similar substances tested in rabbits receiving a cholesterol rich diet decreased LDL oxidation and slowed down the development of atherosclerosis of the aorta (Yamakoshi *et al.*, 1999).

Cellular effects, promising research subjects

It has been recently established that ROS could be mediators in multiple processes regulating gene transcription, showing their actions in phenomena involved in atherosclerotic lesions, including cellular proliferation, maturation and apoptosis (naturally programmed cell death) (Sen and Packer, 1996; Suzuki *et al.*, 1997; Pinkus *et al.*, 1996). The scavenging of ROS by wine polyphenols may have an influence, by a mirror effect, on these processes. However, it is equally possible that the reducing action of polyphenols results in a direct effect on the redox status of the cell and/or nucleus, thus modifying for example the transcription factor AP-1, whose reduced form favours DNA binding (Abate *et al.*, 1990) and the expression of the genes it regulates (for example, there is an AP-1 response element in the DNA regulator domain of glutathion peroxidase). It has also been reported that phenolic acids can increase the expression of *c-fos* and *c-jun* genes (Choi and Moore, 1993). In cells there are ROS sensors-like. For example, ROS interact with the amino terminal kinase of c-Jun (Lo *et al.*, 1996) resulting in an increased phosphorylation of c-Jun and an increased expression of AP-1 transcriptional activity; IkB kinases (Mercurio *et al.*, 1997) lead to alleviate the inhibition of the NF-kB transcriptional activity; both pathways lead to gene expression regulated by transcription factors AP-1 and NF-kB. The process remain to be thoroughly explored. Special attention must be paid to the expression mechanism of genes coding for enzymes involved in the production or destruction of ROS, *i.e.* in the regulation of the redox state of the cell. If the redox status (or antioxidants) regulate gene expression, inversely it is likely that the expression of genes has an effect on the redox status.

The positive action on the LDL vitamin E content due to polyphenols administration could induce protective effects against atherosclerosis resulting from cellular actions of vitamin E on the vascular wall (Nunes *et al.*, 1997) and on monocytes/macrophages (Cachia *et al.*, 1998).

Finally, catechin has also been shown to significantly reduced the progression of aortic lipid strakes in hyperlipidemic hamsters (Xu *et al.*, 1998). It remarkably confirmed that, regardless of the mechanism involved, a beneficial anti-atheromatous effect related to wine consumption can be directly demonstrated. It is worthwhile mentioning that atheroma in this type of animal is generally considered a good model for humans, and more specifically that the amount of catechin added to food during this experiment corresponded to that normally consumed by humans. However, this work should not limit in future the interest of researchers just to the catechin molecule, or only to molecules present in red wine with a flavonoid structure. For example, it was mentioned at the VIIth Entretiens d'Agropolis (Doco *et al.*, UR Biopolymères des Arômes, INRA, Montpellier) that on a strictly nutritional level, wine should not be considered today as a source of chronic lead contamination, not only because of an improved control of potential contamination during the wine making process, but also and mainly because of the presence of complex sugars (rhamnogalacturonane II dimers) in red wine and white wine as well, at concentrations of 50-150 mg/l which possess the capacity of binding to lead (or other toxic cations), thus making them unavailable to the body of the consumer.

Conclusion

Wine (with alcohol or alcohol-free) polyphenols consumed are found in the general circulation and act there as antioxidants – but this is not their only action – thus resulting in different processes that make an action against atherosclerosis plausible. A better knowledge of bioavailability, metabolism and mechanism of action of constitutive molecules of the different wine polyphenol families requires considerable methodological demands. This must lead to a better understanding of the role of wine in cardiovascular prevention and thus avoid purely factual announcements that may result in hasty conclusions. One of the key questions consists in particular to know if there are effects that, in certain cases, could be due not to the substances present in the drink, but to metabolic derivatives or degradation products of these substances appearing in the body. It could especially apply to those that, due to their molecular mass, do not seem able to pass through the intestinal wall, and therefore have a longer residence time within the intestinal lumen and thus be attacked by intestinal microflora. Finally, the difference between the polyphenol contents actually present in plasma (and probably the entire systemic environment), on the one hand, and those most often used *in vitro* by investigators and which are known to be active (especially in terms of antioxidant properties), on the other, shows that we do not have today definitive and totally convincing interpretations to explain biologically the polyphenol effects in terms of cardiovascular prevention. The search for new biological indicators and their use in humans in nutritional intervention that have to be further developped probably will provide a response to the questions that remain unanswered at the moment.

REFERENCES

- Abate C, Patel L, Rauscher FJD. Redox regulation of fos and jun DNA-binding activity *in vitro*. *Science* 1990 ; 249 : 1157-61.

- Abu-Amsha R, Croft KD, Puddley IB, Proudfoot JM, Beilin LJ. Phenolic content of various beverages determines the extent of inhibition of human serum and low-density lipoprotein oxidation *in vitro* : identification and mechanism of action of cinnamic acid derivatives from red wine. *Clin Sci* 1996 ; 91 : 449-58.

- Afanas'ev IB, Dorozhko AI, Brodskii AV, Kostyuk A, Potapovitch AI. Chelating and free radical scavenging mechanims of inhibitory action of rutin and quercetin in lipid peroxidation. *Biochem Pharmacol* 1989 ; 38 : 1763-9.

- Andriambeloson E, Kleschyov AL, Muller B, Beretz A, Stoclet JC, Andriantsitohaina R. Nitric oxide production and endothelium-dependent vasorelaxation induced by wine polyphenols in rat aorta. *Br J Pharmacol* 1997 ; 120 : 1053-8.

- Bedwell S, Dean RT, Jessup W. The action of defined oxygen-centred free radicals on human low-density lipoprotein. *Biochem J* 1989 ; 262 : 707-12.

- Cabanis JC, Cabanis MT, Cheynier V, Teissedre PL. Tables de composition. In : Flanzy C, ed. *Œnologie : fondements scientifiques et technologiques*. Paris : Lavoisier Tec-Doc, 1998 : 316-36.

- Cachia O, Léger CL, Descomps B. Monocyte superoxide production is inversely related to normal content of α-tocopherol in low-density lipoprotein. *Atherosclerosis* 1998 ; 138 : 263-9.

- Cao G, Russell RM, Lischner N, Prior RL. Serum antioxidant capacity is increased by consumption of stawberries, spinach, red wine or vitamin C in elderly women. *J Nutr* 1998 ; 128 : 2383-90.

- Carando S, Teissedre PL, Ferrière M, Descomps B, Cabanis JC. Boissons alcoolisées et cardiopathies ischémiques. *Cah Nutr Diet* 1998a ; 33 : 182-7.

- Carando S, Teissedre PL, Léger C, Cabanis JC. Consommation de vin, bière, spiritueux et maladies cardiovasculaires. *Sci Alim* 1998b ; 18 : 117-27.

- Carbonneau MA, Léger CL, Monnier L, Bonnet C, Michel F, Fouret G, Dedieu F, Descomps B. Supplementation with wine phenolic compounds increases the antioxidant capacity of plasma and vitamin E of low-density lipoprotein without changing the lipoprotein Cu^{2+} - oxidizability ; possible explanation by phenolic location. *Eur J Clin Nutr* 1997 ; 51 : 682-90.

- Carbonneau MA, Léger CL, Senglat C, Fouret G, Monnier L, Descomps B. The *ex vivo* Montpellier's study : role of polyphenol compounds of wine origin given to human volunteers in the antioxidative protection of plasma and low-density lipoprotein. *COST* 1998 ; 916 : 147-52.

- Cartron E, Carbonneau MA, Fouret G, Descomps B, Léger CL. Specific antioxidant activity of caffeoyl derivatives and other natural phenolic compounds : LDL protection against oxidation and decrease in the pro-inflammatory lysophosphatidylcholine production. *J Agr Food Chem* (sous presse).

- Chiu HC, Jeng JR, Shieh SM. Increased oxidizability of plasma low density lipoprotein from patients with coronary artery disease. *Biochim Biophys Acta* 1994 ; 1225 : 200-8.

- Choi HS, Moore DD. Induction of c-fos and c-jun gene expression by phenolic antioxidants. *Mol Endocrinol* 1993 ; 7 : 1596-602.

- Cominacini L, Garbin U, Pastorino AM, Davoli A, Campagnola M, De Santis A, Pasini C, Faccini GB, Trevisan MT, Bertozzo L. Predisposition to LDL oxidation in patients with and without angiographically established coronary artery disease. *Atherosclerosis* 1993 ; 99 : 63-70.

- Darley-Usmar VM, Hohgg N, O'Leary VJ, Wilson MT, Moncada S. The simultaneous generation of superoxide and nitric oxide can initiate lipid peroxidation in human low density lipoprotein. *Free Rad Res Coms* 1992 ; 17 : 9-20.

- Daugherty A, Dunn JL, Rateri DL, Heinecke JW. Myeloperoxidase, a catalyst for lipoprotein oxidation, is expressed in human atherosclerotic lesions. *J Clin Invest* 1994 ; 94 : 437-44.

- Donovan JL, Bell JR, Kasim-Karakas S, German JB, Walsem RL, Hansen RJ, Waterhouse L. Catechin is present as metabolites in human plasma after consumption of red wine. *J Nutr* 1999 ; 129 : 1662-8.

- Duthie GG, Pedersen MW, Gardner PT, Morrice PC, Jenkinson AM, McPhail DB, Steele GM. *Eur J Clin Nutr* 1998 ; 52 : 733-6.

- Fang X, Weintraub NL, Chappell DA, Zwacka RM, Engelhardt JF, Oberley LW, Yan T, Heistad DD, Spector AA. Overexpression of human superoxide dismutase inhibits oxidation of low-density lipoprotein by endothelial cells. *Circ Res* 1998 ; 82 : 1289-97.

- Fernandez MA, Saenz MT, Garcia MD. Anti-inflammatory activity in rats and mice of phenolic acids isolated from Scrophularia frutescens. *J Pharm Pharmacol* 1998 ; 50 : 1183-6.

- Frankel EN, Waterhouse AL, Teissedre PL. Principal phenolic phytochemicals in selected California wines and their antioxidant activity in inhibiting oxidation of human low-density lipoproteins. *J Agric Food Chem* 1995 ; 43 : 890-4.

- Fuhrman B, Lavy A, Aviram M. Consumption of red wine with meals reduces the susceptibility of human plasma and low-density to lipid oxidation. *Am J Clin Nutr* 1995 ; 61 : 549-54.

- Hackett AM, Griffiths LA, Broillet A, Wermeille M. The metabolism and excretion of (+)-[14C]cyanidanol-3 in man following oral administration. *Xenobiotica* 1983 ; 13 : 279-86.

- Hollman PC, de Vries JHM, van Leeuwen SD, Mengelers MJB, Katan MB. Absorption of dietary quercetin glycosides and quercetin in healthy ileostomy volunteers. *Am J Clin Nutr* 1995 ; 62 : 1276-82.

- Hollman PCH. Bioavailability of flavonoids. *Eur J Clin Nutr* 1997 ; 51 (Suppl. 1) : S66-S69.

- Husain SR, Cillard J, Cillard P. Hydroxyl radical scavenging activity of flavonoids. *Phytochem* 1987 ; 26 : 2489-91.

- Kuhn H, Heydeck D, Hugou I, Gnowotta C. In vivo action of 15-lipoxygenase in early stages of human atherosclerosis. *J Clin Incest* 1997 ; 99 : 888-93.

- Lo YYC, Wong JMS, Cruz TF. Reactive oxygen species mediate cytokine activation of c-jun NH2-terminal kinases. *J Biol Chem* 1996 ; 271 : 15703-7.

- Ma XL, Lopez BL, Liu GL, Christopher TA, Gao F, Guo Y, Feuerstein GZ, Ruffolo RR Jr, Barone FC, Yue TL. Hypercholesterolemia impairs a detoxification mechanism against peroxynitrite and renders the vascular tissue more susceptible to oxidative injury. *Circ Res* 1997 ; 80 : 894-901.

- Manach C, Morand C, Crespy V, Démigné C, Texier O, Régérat F, Rémésy C. Quercetin is recovered in human plasma as conjugated derivatives which retain antioxidant properties. *FEBS Letters* 1998 ; 426 : 331-6.

- Maxwell S, Cruickshank A, Thorpe G. Red wine and antioxidant activity in serum. *Lancet* 1994 ; 344 : 193-4.

- Mercurio F, Zhu H, Murray BW, Shevchenko A, Bennett BL, Li J, Young DB, Barbosa M, Mann M, Manning A, Rao A. IKK-1 and IKK-2 : cytokine-activated IkappaB kinases essential for NF-kB activation. *Science* 1997 ; 278 : 860-6.

- Moroney MA, Alcaraz MJ, Foder RA, Carey F, Hoult JRS. Selectivity of neutrophil 5-lipoxygenase and cyclo-oxygenase inhibition by an anti-inflammatory flavanoid glycoside and related aglycone flavonoids. *J Pharm Pharmacol* 1988 ; 40 : 787-92.

- Nigdikar SV, Williams NR, Griffin BA, Howard AN. Consumption of red wine polyphenols reduces the susceptibility of low-density lipoproteins to oxidation in vivo. *Am J Clin Nutr* 1998 ; 68 : 258-65.

- Noroozi M, Angerson WJ, Lean MEJ. Effects of flavonoids and vitamin C on oxidative DNA damage to human lymphocytes. *Am J Clin Nutr* 1998 ; 67 : 1210-8.

- Nunes GL, Robinson K, Kalynych A, King III SB, Sgoutas DS, Berk BC. Vitamin C and E inhibit O_2^- production in the pig coronary artery. *Circulation* 1997 ; 96 : 3593-601.

- Pannala AS, Rice-Evans CA, Halliwell B, Singh S. Inhibition of peroxynitrite-mediated tyrosine nitration by catechin polyphenols. *Biochem Biophys Res Commun* 1997 ; 232 : 164-8.

- Pellegrini N, Pareti FI, Stabile F, Brusamolino A, Simonetti P. Effects of moderate consumption of red wine on platelet aggregation and haemostatic variables in healthy volunteers. *Eur J Clin Nutr* 1996 ; 50 : 209-13.

- Pinkus R, Weiner LM, Danile V. Role of oxidants and antioxidants in the induction of AP-1, NF-kB, and glutathion S-transferase gene expression. *J Biol Chem* 1996 ; 274 : 13422-9.

- Puurunen M, Mantari M, Manninen V, Tenkanen L, Alfthan G, Ehnholm C, Vaarala O, Aho K, Palosuo T. Antibody against oxidised low-density lipoprotein predicting myocardial infarction. *Arch Intern Med* 1994 ; 154 : 2605-9.

- Regnström J, Nilsson J, Tornvall P, Landou C, Hamsten A. Susceptibility to low-density lipoprotein oxidation and coronary atherosclerosis in man. *Lancet* 1992 ; 339 : 1183-6.

- Renaud SC, Guéguen R, Schenker J, d'Houtaud A. Alcohol and mortality in middle-aged men from Eastern France. *Epidemiology* 1998 ; 9 : 184-8.

- Ruf JC, Berger JL, Renaud S. Platelet ebound effect of alcohol withdrawal and wine drinking in rats. *Arterioscler Thromb Vasc Biol* 1995 ; 15 : 140-4.

- Salonen JT, Ylä-Herttuala S, Yamamoto R, Butler S, Korpela H, Salonen R. Autoantibody against oxidised LDL and progression of carotid atherosclerosis. *Lancet* 1992 ; 339 : 883-7.

- Savenkova MI, Mueller DM, Heinecke JW. Tyrosyl radical generated by myeloperoxidase is a physiological catalyst for the initiation of lipid peroxidation in low density lipoprotein. *J Biol Chem* 1994 ; 269 : 20394-400.

- Sen CK, Packer L. Antioxidant and redox regulation of gene transcription. *FASEB J* 1996 ; 10 : 709-20.

- Serafini M, Maiani G, Ferro-Luzzi A. Alcohol-free red wine enhances plasma antioxidant capacity in humans. *J Nutr* 1998 ; 128 : 1003-7.

- Steinbrecher UP, Zhang H, Lougheed M. Role of oxidatively modified LDL in atherosclerosis. *Free Rad Biol Med* 1990 ; 9 : 155-68.

- Suzuki YJ, Forman HJ, Sevanian A. Oxidants as stimulators of signal transduction. *Free Rad Biol Med* 1997 ; 22 : 269-85.

- Tebib K, Besançon P, Rouanet JM. Dietary grape seed tannins affect lipoproteins, lipoprotein lipases and tissue lipids in rats fed hypercholesterolemic diets. *J Nutr* 1994 ; 124 : 2451-7.

- Tebib K, Rouanet JM, Besançon P. Antioxidant effects of dietary polymeric grape seed tannins in tissues of rats fed a high cholesterol-vitamin E-deficient diet. *Food Chem* 1997 ; 59 : 135-41.

- Teissedre PL, Frankel EN, Waterhouse AL, Peleg H, German JB. Inhibition of *in vitro* human LDL oxidation by phenolic antioxidants from grapes and wines. *J Sci Food Agric* 1996 ; 70 : 55-61.

- Torel J, Cillard J, Cillard P. Antioxidant activity of flavonoids and reactivity with peroxy radical. *Phytochem* 1986 ; 25 : 383-5.

- Viana M, Barbas C, Bonet B, Bonet MV, Castro M, Fraile MV, Herrera E. In vitro effects of a flavonoid-rich extract on LDL oxidation. *Atherosclerosis* 1996 ; 123 : 83-91.

- Wever RMF, Lüscher TF, Cosentino F, Rabelink TJ. Atherosclerosis and the two faces of endothelial nitric oxide synthase. *Circulation* 1998 ; 97 : 108-12.

- Whitehead TP, Robinson D, Allaway S, Syms J, Hale A. Effect of red wine ingestion on the antioxidant capacity of serum. *Clin Chem* 1995 ; 41 : 32-5.

- Wollfram S, Weber T, Grenacher B, Scharrer A. A Na^+ dependent mechanism is involved in mucosal uptake of connamic acid across the jejunal brush border in rats. *J Nutr* 1995 ; 125 : 1300-8.

- Woodford FP, Whitehead TP. Is measuring serum antioxidant capacity clinically useful ? *Ann Clin Biochem* 1998 ; 35 : 48-56.

- Wu R, Nityanand S, Berglund L, Lithell H, Holm G, Lefvert AK. Antibodies against cardiolipin and oxidatively modified LDL in 50-year-old men predict myocardial infarction. *Arterioscler Thromb Vasc Biol* 1997 ; 17 : 3159-63.

- Xu R, Yokoyama WH, Irving D, Rein D, Walzem RL, German JB. Effect of dietary catechin and vitamin E on aortic fatty streak accumulation in hypercholesterolemuc hamsters. *Atherosclerosis* 1998 ; 137 : 29-36.

- Yamakoshi J, Kataoka S, Koga T, Ariga T. Proanthocyanidin-rich extract from grape seeds attenuates the development of aortic atherosclerosis in cholesterol-fed rabbits. *Atherosclerosis* 1999 ; 142 : 139-49.

- Ylä-Herttuala S. Is oxidized low-density lipoprotein present *in vivo* ? *Curr Opin Lipidol* 1998 ; 9 : 337-44.

Beneficial effects of fruits and vegetables on health

Pierre Besançon

Thousands of years ago fruits and vegetables, along with the first cultivated cereals, were already at the core of the diet of the early Mediterranean civilisations. Currently, it has been recognised that increased consumption of fruits and vegetables constitutes, on the one hand, an obvious asset for a good nutritional balance, and provides on the other hand an undeniable health benefit.

Epidemiological studies (*see chapter* "Health benefits of Mediterranean consumption model") clearly demonstrate the essential role of fruits and vegetables in the prevention of numerous chronic pathologies; cancers and cardiovascular diseases.

Starting with the average hypothesis of a fruit and vegetable consumption of the order of 350 g/day, *i.e.* approximately 150 g/1,000 kcal, major daily and especially interindividual variations must be envisaged. According to Law and Morris (1998), the ischaemic vascular risk decreases by 15% when one goes from the 10 percentile of the population consuming the least amount of fruit and vegetables to the groups above the 90 percentile corresponding to the greatest fruit and vegetable consumption, *i.e.* approximately 600 g/day. Between these two extremes, fruit consumption is multiplied by 4 and that of vegetables by 2. With respect to the prevention of some forms of cancer, many reviews confirm the preventive or protective effect of fruits and vegetables (Tavani and La Vecchia, 1995; Schliengler *et al.*, 1998).

The words fruit and vegetable cover an extremely wide variety of food products consumed raw or cooked and fresh or dried, from very different parts of plants, which are themselves from numerous botanical families. This can be (Come and Corbineau, 1999) entire plantlets (soybean sprout, radish sprout), stems (asparagus), whole leaves (cabbage, watercress, spinach, parsley, dandelion, lettuce), leaf bases (leeks), petioles (celery, fennel, rhubarb), buds (Brussels sprouts, endives), inflorescences (artichokes, broccoli, cauliflower), seeds (pulses), roots (beetroot, carrot, turnip, radish), bulbs (garlic, onion), tubers (potato), rhizomes (ginger), carpophores (mushrooms). Fruits are consumed as berries or drupes, or as vegetables: these can be fleshy (aubergine, cucumber, pumpkin, hot pepper, sweet pepper, tomato) or dry fruits (cereal grains, chestnut, walnut, hazelnut, kidney bean pods, sweet corn). This botanical and anatomical diversity makes that fruits and vegetables include food products with an extremely varied nutritional value; from the point of view of the nutrionist it is their combination that constitutes their wealth. On the other hand, the monotone consumption of a single type of product would be a nutritional mistake.

In general, they are water rich products, with a low energetic value and high nutritional density, rich in minerals, vitamins, fibres and various other compounds that are biologically active but are not really considered as nutrients; the antioxidants and phyto-oestrogens. However, pulses and grains are characterised by low water content, high complex carbohydrates, fibres and sometimes lipids content. The case of pulses from the leguminous family merits special attention due to their high proteins, fibres and minerals content (Besançon, 1978), but also antinutritional factors. Legume seeds, which are often rejected, should be rehabilitated in the balance of the diet along with fresh vegetables.

The mechanisms invoked to explain the health benefit of fruits and vegetables involve very different properties:
– antioxidant properties (vitamins, polyphenols);
– action on the intestinal bacterial flora (fibres);
– regulation of detoxification enzymes (antioxidants);
– inhibition of formation of carcinogenic compounds (fibres);
– specific effects of hormone (phyto-oestrogens) or immune (phenolic compounds) nature;
– mechanical action on the digestive tract (fibres).

VITAMINS

Vitamin requirements may be largely covered by fruits and vegetables, sometimes they are the almost exclusive source, as is the case of vitamin C and folic acid. On the other hand, an exclusively vegetarian diet would not cover adequately some vitamin requirements, as in the case of vitamin B12.

The mechanisms of action and the effects of vitamins have been largely described elsewhere. Very schematically and overall, it can be considered that:
– water soluble vitamins of the B group (vitamin B1 or thiamine, vitamin B2 or riboflavin, vitamin B3 or PP or niacin, vitamin B6 or pyridoxine, vitamin B9 or folic acid, etc.) behave as enzymatic cofactors in many metabolic enzymatic systems,
– fat soluble vitamins (vitamin A or retinol, vitamin D3 or cholecalciferol) as effectors at a cellular and nucleic level, acting on protein synthesis and cellular differentiation,
– antioxidant properties are shared between vitamin C (ascorbic acid), vitamin E (α-tocopherol), carotenoids and in particular β-carotene, a vitamin A precursor,
– vitamin E regulates also some cellular mechanisms.

As an example, it should be remembered (*see chapters* "Olive oil, olive oil by-products and olive fruit: current data and developments concerning the food and health relationship" and "Wine consumption and cardiovascular disease prevention") that β-carotene and vitamin C, abundant in fruits and vegetables, can be considered as protectors of the vitamin E found in membranes and especially in low density lipoproteins (LDL), which leads to a reduction in the risk of lipid peroxidation of the lipoproteins and cellular membranes.

Another example concerns folic acid, particularly abundant in green vegetables. Vitamin B9 (folic acid) and vitamin B12 control transmethylation reactions in metabolism. Folate deficiency results in an increase in homocysteine, a methionine synthesis precursor, or on the contrary, a product of methionine demethylation. It is known that an increase in homocysteinemia is correlated with an increased vascular risk. Furthermore, the teratogenic effects on the neural tube related to folic acid deficiency during pregnancy are also known. The level of folate consumption is sometimes considered as marginal by some in occidental populations and specifically in some women; this can be easily solved by an increase in the consumption of green vegetable and certain fruits (orange) (Kushi et al., 1995).

The efficiency of various micronutrients, and especially vitamins, seems to depend on two factors: their bioavailability and synergic effects. In order to explain the bioavailability variations, the physico-chemical form of the molecules and their biochemical environment that have influence on digestibility and absorption, may be evoked. Folates are less effective than folic acid to restore a normal homocysteine plasma level (Law and Morris, 1998). Furthermore, bioavailability can also depend on physiological factors, such as the age of the subjects (Borel et al., 1997, Borel et al., 1998).

OTHER ANTIOXIDANTS

Apart from the antioxydant vitamins (ascorbic acid, tocopherol, retinol) many other plant micro constituents have been classified in plants for their antioxidant properties:
- carotenoids, which are not retinol precursors: α-carotene, tomato lycopene, onion β-cryptaxanthine, green vegetable luteine;
- phenolic compounds: phenolic acids, phenolic alcohols and flavonoids;
- sulphur compounds: allyl sulphide (garlic, onion);
- terpenes: limonene in citrus fruit;
- and to a lesser extent, isothiocyanates of some leguminous plants and glucosinates from cruciferae.

Phenolic compounds can be classified as a function of their chemical structure (Macheix and Fleuriet, 1999) *(Table I)*.

Phenolic compounds play many roles in plants as well as in fruits and vegetables which are issued from these plants after harvest: colour, bitterness, astringency, antioxidant properties. These compounds are involved in enzymatic browning phenomena (Billot, 1999), which generally lead to a deterioration of the organoleptic and nutritional qualities.

The mode of action of all these antioxidant compounds are situated at different levels:
- as reducing agents or antioxidants, strictly speaking: protection of vitamin E and indirectly lipoperoxidation, in particular in membranes and LDL;
- as free radical scavengers, during phase I of detoxification mechanisms, especially producing the superoxide anion;
- as chelators of metals (iron, copper) involved in oxidation phenomena;
- as inhibitors of certain enzymes: lipoxygenase, cyclooxygenase;
- as activators of phase II detoxification mechanism: glutathion-S-transferase.

Specific effects must be added: antiviral or immunomodulators (certain flavonoids), antiproliferative (certain phenolic alcohols). Finally the antioxidant effects of flavonoids explain their DNA protection role against oxidation related the mutagenesis risks.

Many of these properties depend on the bioavailability of the micro constituents involved, some of which have large molecular weights. It is not easy to understand why tannin oligomers are effective *in vivo* while only monomeric type flavonoids (catechin) seem to really go through the intestinal barrier (results of the laboratories GBSA-nutrition and Human Nutrition and Atherogenesis, Montpellier) (*see also chapter* "Wine consumption and cardiovascular disease prevention"). Therefore, there are also specific effects that are locally manifested on the digestive mucosa.

Table I. Classification of some phenolic compounds

Number of carbons	Carbon skeleton	Polyphenol class and examples	
7	C6-C1	Phenolic acids of the benzoic series	Gallic acid, protocatechic acid, parahydroxybenzoic acid, vanillic acid
9	C6-C3	Phenolic acids of the cinnamic series	Caffeic acid, chlorogenic acid, sinapic acid, paracoumaric acid (coumarin: lactone derivative)
9	C6-C3	Phenolic alcohols	(Hydroxy)tyrosol
15	C6-C3-C6	Flavonoids	Catechin flavonols, Procyanidines, Quercetin, rutin, kaempferol flavonols, Delphinidine anthocyanes
		Isoflavones	Genistein, daidzin
N	(C15)n	Tannins	More or less polymerised and more or less galloylated (gallic acid) flavonoids
N	(C6-C3)n	Lignin	(cf. fibres)

MINERALS

Fruits and vegetables are an important source of many mineral elements; their respective richness is a specific characteristic of each product and may also depend on the production and transformation conditions. The CIQUAL composition tables provide detailed information. Special mention may be made concerning potassium and sodium. Fruits and vegetables are always a good source of potassium and provide very small amounts of sodium, which, in view of the roles of these elements on the regulation of intra- and extracellular osmotic balance, is an additional argument to explain the beneficial role of fruits and vegetables in the prevention of high blood pressure and thus vascular complications. Another example is that of selenium, present in particular in cereals and some vegetables, which plays an important role in the body's defence as a constitutive element of selenium-dependent glutathionperoxydase, which is itself one of the key enzymes in the protection metabolism against oxidative stress.

Finally it must be mentioned that the bioavailability of mineral elements is largely conditioned by the presence of other food factors. Vitamin C intake as well as a good balance of amino acids, especially lysine, conditions to a large extent the absorption of iron. On the other hand, phytates, abundant in grains from leguminous plants and unrefined whole cereals, reduce the absorption of bivalent cations such as calcium, magnesium, iron, zinc by complexing them. Also the phosphorus present as phytate or phytic acid (myoinositol hexaphosphate) is not very available. Some organic acids (oxalic acid) can also play a negative role.

PHYTO-OESTROGENS

Phyto-oestrogens, which behave as oestrogen analogues, include several different molecules: isoflavones as well as lignans and coumestanes. They are found in plants from the leguminous family and especially in soy bean, but also in other pulses (lentils, chickpeas, etc.). Phyto-oestrogens are either under the aglycone (genistein, daidzein) form or under a glycosylated, acetylated and malonylated form. After ingestion phyto-oestrogens are not degraded in the stomach and the small intestine; they can be biotransformed by colon bacteria: glucuronidase producing bacteria deconjugate them and thus favour faecal elimination. The best absorbed form is in general glycosylated. An enterohepatic cycle of phyto-oestrogen allows an increase in their plasma concentrations to levels above those of endogenous oestrogens. Their effects are varied and depend in particular on their affinity for oestrogenic receptors (*see part* "Epidemiology"). They have a diuretic effect, they increase bone mass by inhibiting osteoclastic bone resorption. A reduction in blood lipids and more specifically LDL-cholesterol, by the action of phyto-oestrogens has been observed. Finally, like all flavonoids they show antioxidant properties. Effects on cellular proliferation have also been reported. Conjugated daidzein is more effective than genistein, probably due to a better stability within the intestinal lumen. These compounds benefit from renewed interest, in view of the beneficial effect attributed to them with respect to protection against oxidation stress but mainly against carcinogenesis mechanisms (Setchell, 1998).

FIBRES

Since 1974, date when Trowell and Burkitt formulated the "fibre hypothesis", fibres are defined as plant cell residues not attacked by digestive enzymes in humans. Dietary fibres are essentially composed of complex polyholosides (cellulose, hemicellulose, pectins, gums) and polyphenols (lignin). Due to their localisation in plants, fibres are also associated with numerous other substances (see *Table II*, adapted from Schweizer, 1986 and *Table III*).

Table II. Classification of fibres and associated substances

Non carbohydrate compounds	{ Proteins, Cutin, Waxes, Silica, Phytates	} Compounds associated with plant walls
	LIGNIN	} Compounds associated with fibres
Non starch carbohydrate compounds	{ CELLULOSE, HEMICELLULOSES, PECTINS, Gums, Mucilage, Algae and micro-organism polysaccharides	} "Dietary fibres"

Due to the diversity and complexity of the chemical structure of fibres *(Table III)*, numerous analytical methods proposed are often little specific and lead to very divergent results. The old method to determine gross cellulose, also called Weende cellulose, resulted in greatly underestimated fibre contents; numerous food composition tables are still based on such results. The most recent methods differentiate:

– insoluble fibres: cellulose, hemicellulose, lignin,

– soluble fibres: pectins, gums, certain hemicelluloses (low molecular weight).

The soluble fibres + insoluble fibres sum constitutes the "Total Dietary Fibre" entity (*see technical note*: "Dietary fibres: nutritional interest in human diet").

The diversity of dietary fibres makes them compounds with extremely varied modes of action. Overall, fibres are the only "nutrients" which act as such because they cannot be digested in the human digestive tract and monogastric animals. Only some fibres can be fermented, thus attacked by micro-organisms in the colon. However, polygastric ruminants degrade and ferment fibres in the rumen.

Due to the absence of hydrolysis by physiological enzymes and their capacity to bind water (cellulose, hemicelluloses), fibres contribute to increasing digestive volume, which tends to regularise transit by slowing down gastric emptying and stimulating intestinal motricity. When the fibres cannot be fermented in the colon, they also contribute to increasing faecal volume. On the contrary, fermentable fibres (pectin, gums, certain hemicelluloses) become the substrate of the colon flora that in its development promotes an acid fermentation and the production of very short chain volatile fatty acids (acetate, butyrate), which contribute to decreasing the pH; under certain conditions butyrate has been attributed with tumour cell proliferation reduction properties. The colon fermentation metabolism is regulated by numerous factors and it is believed that in the presence of fermentable fibres the growth of glucuronidase secreting bacteria is reduced. This is followed by a decrease in the deconjugation of phyto-oestrogens, with, as a consequence, a facilitated absorption.

Table III. Chemical structure of fibres

Class of fibres	Carbohydrates of the main chain / Types of bonds	Secondary chains
Cellulose	Glucose β1-4	
Hemicellulose	Xylanes: xylose β1-4 β-glucans: glucose β1-4, β1-3 Mannans: mannose β1-4 Galactans: galactose β1-4, β1-6 Glucomannans: glucose, mannose β1-4 Arabinogalactans: β1-3, β1-6	Glucuronic acid Arabinose Glucose Xylose
Pectins	Galacturonans: galacturonic acid β1-4 more or less methylated Arabinogalactans: galactose and arabinose β1-4, β1-5	Galactose Arabinose Rhamnose Galacturonic acid more or less methylated
Gums	Glucuronic acid and galacturonic acid β1-4 Mannose β1-4	Arabinose Xylose Mannose Galacturonic acid
Mucilage	Galaturonic acid β1-4	(cf. pectins)
Agarose	Galactose β1-4	
Carrhagenans	Id. agarose + sulphate + cation (carrhagenates)	
Alginates	Mannuronic acid and galacturonic acid β1-4	
Xanthanes	Glucose β1-4 Mannose (acetylated) Glucuronic acid	
Lignin	Phenylpropane	

Another aspect of the effects of fibres is related to their capacity to adsorb other components, or even form complexes. This effect is considered as fairly favourable if one considers biliary salts: the latter are fixed, preferentially eliminated by faecal route, thus reducing the possibility of their biotransformation in carcinogenic compounds. We have also mentioned the inhibitory action of fibres on primary biliary salt dehydroxylation into secondary biliary salts.

On the contrary, the cation (calcium, iron, zinc, etc.) binding capacity of fibres (fibres rich in uronic acid, pectins, acid hemicelluloses) can reduce availability. Also, the presence of fibres can lead to a reduction in the activity of certain digestive enzymes. However, these phenomena are often equally due to the presence of true enzyme inhibitors, present in leguminous pulses and in whole cereals: protein inhibitors and phytates. Condensed lignin and tannins also share with carbohydrate type fibres the property of forming more or less strong bonds with proteins or enzymes, thus behaving like enzyme inhibitors.

Apart from the digestive effects (acceleration of intestinal transit, colic fermentation modulation), fibres have indirect effects on metabolism: decrease of postprandial glycaemia and insulinemia, reduction of carbohydrate glycaemic index, improvement of lipid metabolism parameters: postprandial lipemia, cholesterol (Lairon, 1990).

Fruits and vegetables, unrefined cereals and leguminous pulses constitute essential fibre sources. Soluble fibres that are considered as a bit more abundant in cereals have a preponderant effect on colic fermentation and metabolic effects (lipids). By definition insoluble fibres have a primordial role on the regulation of digestive transit. The ingestion of total fibres is currently less than 20 g/day: it should be greatly increased both in the form of cereals and as fruits and vegetables.

Macronutrients: proteins, carbohydrates, lipids

Fruits and vegetables contain little protein, except rare cases; the lipids which are also present in small amounts are fairly rich in monounsaturated and polyunsaturated fatty acids, possibly protected from oxidation by the presence of antioxidants. The carbohydrates present in fruits and vegetables are quite diverse: they are represented by soluble carbohydrates with intermediate sweetening strength (glucose: 0.7 and fructose: 1.3). The presence of polyols (alcohol sugars, such as sorbitol) in certain fruits gives them a sweet taste (sweetening strength 0.6 to 1.0) while reducing the energetic density, as polyols are not digested; on the other hand they can be fermented and generate short chain fatty acids by fermentation. In leguminous plants oligosides are found which are not very digestible but can be fermented; most of them are α-galactosides (raffinose, stachyose, etc.): they thus contribute to reinforce the "fibre" effect of pulses and beans.

Proteins are abundant (20 to 30%) in legume seeds, while not very abundant in fruits and vegetables; these proteins have the advantage of being relatively well balanced in essential amino acids; they are particularly rich in lysine but poor in sulphur amino acids (methionine, cysteine), as in soybean which makes them complementary to cereal proteins, which are lysine poor. The consumption of legume seeds comes up against the presence of antinutritional factors: fortunately most of them can be easily eliminated or inactivated by the appropriate treatments, especially by thermal denaturation (Besançon, 1995).

Conclusion

It is obvious that fruits and vegetables represent a real health benefit in diet. The epidemiological data are convincing and the mechanisms involved have been demonstrated most of the time. A double challenge remains: the problem of bioavailability of micro constituents involved and synergic effects. Both aspects merit to be developed to validate a number of hypotheses.

Finally, we could finish with a more historical reminder concerning vitamin C, whose role in collagen hydroxylation and support tissue and vascular walls integrity phenomena is well-known. Severe deficiency, known as scurvy, is observed as capillary fragility and bleeding. According to tradition vitamin C is perhaps one of the major winners of the battle of Trafalgar in 1805. Vitamin C probably saved the Royal Navy sailors from scurvy because it was provided by the oranges taken on board the ships on Nelson's orders, while Napoleon's sailors, weakened or decimated by scurvy, while cruising off Spain, were not yet following a Mediterranean diet due to lack of fruits and citrus fruits!

REFERENCES

- Adragna-Bourgeois O, Bourgeois CM. Valeur nutritionnelle des légumes. In : Tirilly Y, Bourgeois CM, eds. *Technologie des légumes*. Paris : Tec et Doc Lavoisier, 1999 : 499-512.

- Besançon P. La valeur nutritionnelle des légumes secs et des protéines de légumineuses. *Rev Fr Diétét* 1978 ; 34 : 5-17.

- Besançon P. Les facteurs antinutritionnels présents dans les graines de légumineuses. Colloque Institut Français de Nutrition, Paris, 1995 : 21-9.

- Billot J. Le brunissement enzymatique. In : Tirilly Y, Bourgeois CM, eds. *Technologie des légumes*. Paris : Tec et Doc Lavoisier, 1999 : 225-46.

- Borel P, Mekki N, Boirie Y. Postprandial chylomicron and plasma vitamin E responses in healthy older subjects compared with younger ones. *Eur J Clin Nutr* 1997 ; 27 : 812-21.

- Borel P, Tyssandier V, Mekki N. Chylomicron β-carotène and retinylalmitate responses are dramatically diminished when men ingest β-carotène with medium-chain triglycerides instead of long-chain triglycerides. *J Nutr* 1998 ; 128 : 1361-7.

- Come D, Corbineau F. Classification et caractéristiques physiologiques majeures des légumes. In : Tirilly Y, Bourgeois CM, eds. *Technologie des légumes*. Paris : Tec et Doc Lavoisier, 1999 : 3-14.

- Kushi LH, Lenart EB, Willett WC. Health implications of Mediterranean diets in light of contemporary knowledge. 1. Plant foods and dairy products. *Am J Clin Nutr* 1995 ; 61 (Suppl.) : 14075-155.

- Lairon D. Les fibres alimentaires. *La Recherche* 1990 ; 21 : 284-92.

- Law MR, Morris JK. By how much does fruit and vegetable consumption reduce the risk of ischaemic heart disease ? *Eur J Clin Nutr* 1998 ; 52 : 549-56.

- Macheix JJ, Fleuriet A. Phenolic compounds in food, enzymatic browning and antioxidative properties. In : Kozlowska H, Fornal J, Zdunczyk Z, eds. *Bioactive substances in food of plant origin*. Vol 1, 97-113.

- Setchell KDR. Phytooestrogenes : the biochemistry, physiology and implications for human health of soy isoflavones. *Am J Clin Nutr* 1998 ; 68 (Suppl.) : 13335-465.

- Schliengler H, Pradignac A, Boichot G, Simon C. Régime végétarien et cancer. *Cah Nutr Diet* 1998 ; 33(2) : 83-8.

- Schweizer TF. Dietary fibers. In : Amado R, Schweizer TF, eds. *Methoden zur bestimmung von natrungfasern*. Londres : Academic Press, 1986 : 53-73.

- Tavani A, La Vecchia C. Fruit and vegetable consumption and cancer risk in a Mediterranean population. *Am J Clin Nutr* 1995 ; 61 (Suppl.) : 13745-75.

Technical information

The nutritional benefit of food is related to certain of their components, specific or not, as we have seen in the previous chapters. Thus, the health benefit of the Mediterranean dietary model results from the ingestion of food in optimal proportions, in order to provide the body of the consumer with components that are essential to health.

Among these components more especially represented in foods from the "Mediterranean model", we will mention polyphenols and fibres, subjects of the following notes, which will mention the main sources in which they are found.

Polyphenols: an introduction

Claude-Louis Léger, Marie-Josephe Amiot-Carlin

Recent publications have reviewed the role of phenolic compounds, which constitute a main dietary intake among antioxydant present in plant-derived foods (Bravo, 1998; Lairon and Amiot, 1999). More recently, some specific data are available on grapes and wine (Cheynier *et al.*, 1998) and olives (Servili *et al.*, 1998).

Table I. Quantity (in mg) of total polyphenol found in various foods

Orange juice (1 glass)	100-2,000	Onion (100 g fresh)	100-2,000
Red wine (1 glass)	100-400 (except. 600)	Legumes (100 g dry)	30-1,700
Coffee (1 cup)	100-300	Berries (100 g fresh)	50-1,200
Tea (1 cup)	150-200	1 apple	30-300
White wine (1 glass)	20-30	1 peach	10-150
Beer (1 glass)	20-30	Tomato (100 g fresh)	85-130
Olive oil (1 spoon)	≤ 6	Olive (100 g fresh)	100-7,000

The contents in total polyphenols of various foods and beverages are reported in *Table I*. It appears that the dietary intake in polyphenols greatly varies according the way of consumption (probably from 0.1 to 10 g per day). Polyphenols are substances coming from the secondary metabolism of plants and represented more than 8,000 different chemical structures. This large class of phytochemicals can be divided in sub-classes of structures with different molecular weights: from small, such as phenolic acids, to high, such as tannins resulting from the condensation of numerous phenolic units. In 1989, Harborne proposed a classification of phenolic compounds in 10 main sub-classes based on their carbon skeleton. Among these 10 sub-classes, the major one is the family of flavonoids, largely represented in fruits and vegetables. Flavonoids with a common skeleton C_6-C_3-C_6 is also divided in different groups corresponding to a different degree of oxidation of the heterocycle C_3: flavanols such as catechin, flavonols such as quercetin, flavones, such as luteolin, flavanones such as hesperidin, anthocyanins such as malvidin and isoflavones such as daidzein and genistein. Isoflavones are also called phytoestrogens or dietary estrogens. Phenolic acids can be divided in two series: the benzoic one with gallic and protocatechuic acids, and the cinnamic serie with caffeic, ferulic and *para*-coumaric acids and their conjugated forms such as caftaric, chlorogenic acids and verbascoside. In addition to these phenolic acids, which are also abundant in numerous plant food products, specific structures can be added coming from olives and olive oil, tyrosol and hydrotyrosol as free or conjugated to elenolic acid, and from wine resveratrol, which is a stilbene corresponding to a di-benzenic structure. As previously reported, some structures correspond to molecules with a high molecular weight. Tannins are one of the major groups of polymers, which are known to participate to astringency, especially in unripe fruits. Tannins are divided in two groups: (1) hydrosable tannins with gallotannins and ellagitannins, and (2) condensed tannins or procyanidins resulting from the condensation of the two main flavanol basic structures that are catechin and epicatechin. Generally, flavonoids, except flavanols, are bound to glycosides. They are called conjugated forms. These glycosides can be acylated with acids including phenolic acids leading to more complex structures found in the class of anthocyanins. Acylation confers to anthocyanins greater colour stability. The contribution of the major different sub-classes of polyphenols to various foods and beverages is given in *Table II*.

Table II. Phenolic compounds and dietary origin

Phenolic classes	Dietary source
Flavonols Flavanones Flavones	Fruits and vegetables
Isoflavones	Legumes
Flavanols	Red wines
Anthocyanins	Red fruits
Proanthocyanidins (or procyanidins)	Red wines, fruits
Phenolic acids/alcohols and derivatives	White and red wines, fruits (including olives), vegetables

In *figure 1* are reported the most common basic phenolic structures. This figure illustrates the chemical diversity of this large class of polyphenols leading to a multiplicity of methodologies (extraction, separation, and detection) to set up for the qualitative and quantitative analysis of each compound, the structure of which corresponds to a specific biological effect. It can be stressed that the determination of total polyphenols only has a relative significance in terms of analysis, biological properties and consequently in terms of nutrition.

Flavonoid type phenolic compounds

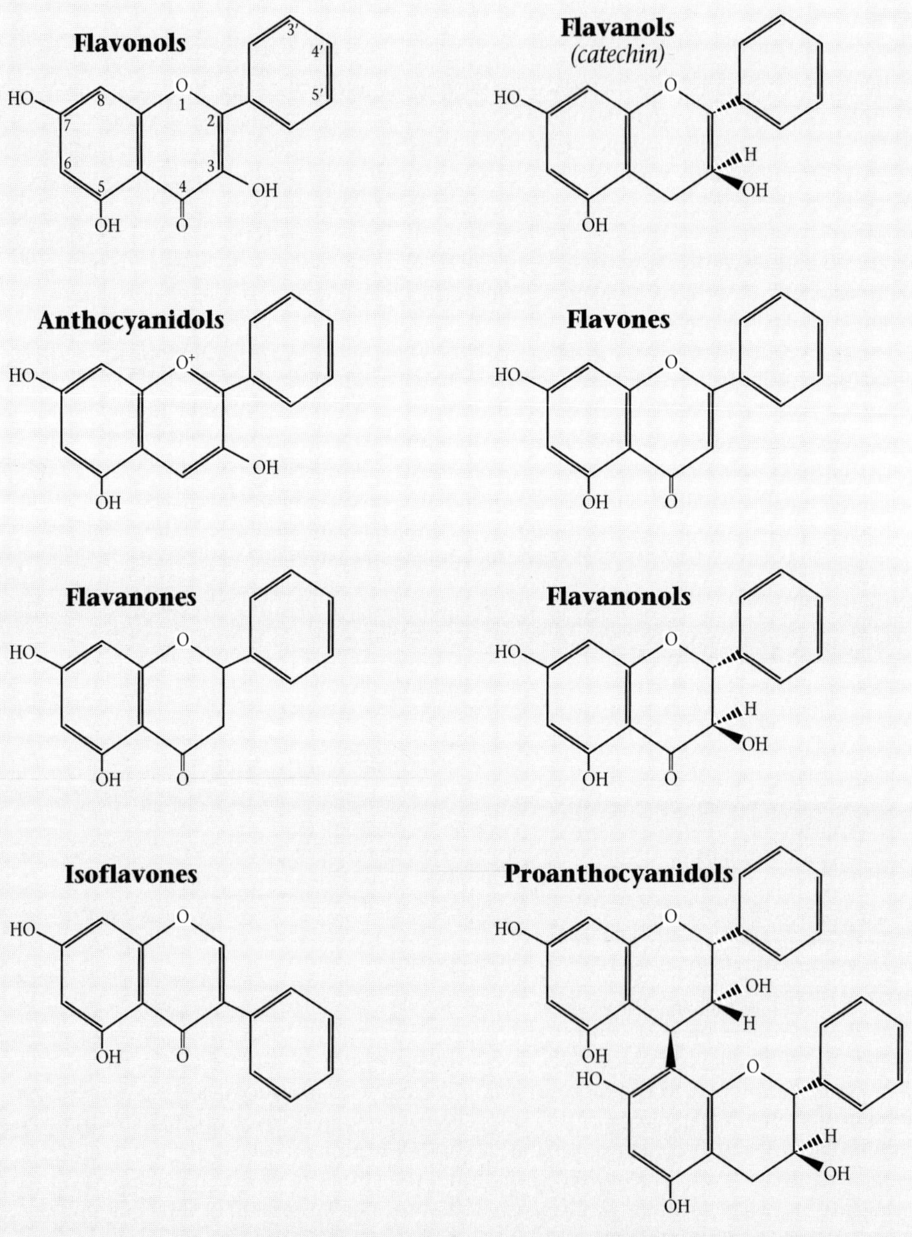

Flavonols

Flavanols *(catechin)*

Anthocyanidols

Flavones

Flavanones

Flavanonols

Isoflavones

Proanthocyanidols

Figure 1. Chemical structures of the main phenolic classes-flavonoid type and non-flavonoid type- In flavonoid structures, substitution (s) with hydroxyle (OH) or methoxyle (OCH_3) can occur on C3', C4' and/or C5'. Flavonoids are frequently glycosylated on C3. For other phenolic compounds, it is indicated with G letter.

Non-flavonoid type phenolic compounds

Gallic acid: benzene ring with OH (top), HO and OH (ortho positions), COOH (para).

Protocachetic acid: benzene ring with OH, OH (ortho), COOH (para).

Caffeic acid: benzene ring with OH, OH (ortho), CH=CH–COOH (para).

Ferulic acid: benzene ring with OH, OCH₃, CH=CH–COOH.

Sinapic acid: benzene ring with OH, two OCH₃ groups, CH=CH–COOH.

Hydroxytyrosol: benzene ring with OH, OH, CH₂–CH₂–OH.

Tyrosol: benzene ring with OH and CH₂–CH₂–OH.

Oleuropein: complex structure with H₃C–OOC, CH₂–COO–CH₂–CH₂– linked to a dihydroxyphenyl ring, CH–CH₃, O–G, pyran ring.

Verbascoside: dihydroxyphenyl–CH=CH–COO–sugar(CH₂OH, OH)–O–CH₂–CH₂–dihydroxyphenyl.

Trans stilbene (Resveratrol): 3,5-dihydroxyphenyl–CH=CH–4-hydroxyphenyl.

References

- Bravo L. Polyphenols : chemistry, dietary sources, metabolism, and nutritional significance. *Nutr Rev* 1998 ; 56 : 317-33.

- Cheynier V, Moutounet M, Sarni-Manchado P. *Œnologie : fondements scientifiques et technologiques*. Paris, Londres, New York, Tec-Doc, 1998.

- Harborne JB. Methods in plant biochemistry, In : *Plant phenolics*. London : Academic Press, 1989.

- Lairon D, Amiot MJ. Flavonoids in food and natural antioxidants in wine. *Curr Opin Lipidol* 1999 ; 10 : 23-8.

- Romani A, Mulinacci N, Pinelli P, Vincieri FF, Cimato A. Polyphenolic content in five tuscany cultivars of *Olea europaea* L.J. *Agric Food Chem* 1999 ; 47 : 964-7.

- Servili M, Bardioloi M, Mariotti F, Montedoro GF. Proceedings of the world conferenceon oilseed and edible oil processing. Vol. 2 : Advances in oils and Fats, antioxidants, and oilseed by-products. AOCS Press, Champaign, Illinois, pp. 289-295, 1998.

Food fibre: nutritional interest in human diet

Denis Lairon

Traditional Mediterranean diet is rich in fibres. In fact the ingestion of dietary fibre has considerably decreased since the beginning of the century due to the intensification in the refining of cereals and the changes in dietary habits in industrialised countries: especially, the decrease in the consumption of cereals and pulses. In France, average fibre ingestion was approximately 31 g/day in 1920; it is of the order of 16 to 17 g/day today. In countries where the population has kept a traditional diet, ingestion levels are clearly higher (30 to 40 g/day).

Dietary fibres are food constituents that are not degraded in the stomach and the small intestine in humans. From a chemical and physico-chemical point of view dietary fibres are a very heterogeneous group. Dietary fibres are polysaccharides, except for lignin, as shown in the *Table* presented in the chapter "Beneficial effects of fruits and vegetables on health".

The complexity of the fibre determination is due to the wide chemical heterogeneity of various components. The current international reference method is the AOAC method (1984 and 1986) that measures fibres as "total dietary fibre" (TDF), as well as soluble and insoluble fibres.

In the diet of Mediterranean zones, the main sources of dietary fibre are unrefined soft wheat (bread, pizza, pastries, etc.) or hard wheat based cereals (pasta, semolina, couscous), peripheral fractions of cereal grains (bran and germ), pulses (chickpeas, beans, lentils, broad beans, etc.), vegetables and fruits. *Table I* shows the total dietary fibre contents of certain foods.

Even if all the mechanisms of action of fibres have not yet been elucidated, there are numerous highly convincing proofs demonstrating that fibres act in a favourable sense on health maintenance.

Among the numerous physiological effects of dietary fibres, the effects on digestive transit and constipation are well-documented. The regulator effects of dietary fibres on the physiology of the colon could improve certain pathological situations. Furthermore, a certain number of data plead in favour of a protective role with respect to cancer of the colon.

Table I. Principal sources of dietary fibres

Food sources of dietary fibres	Content (total fibres, AOAC method)	
	g/100 g	Fresh matter
Wheat bran		40-45
Oat bran*	16-25	
Almonds*		13-15
Whole wheat bread		7-8
White, red beans, cooked*	7-9	
Dry figs*	7-8	
Prunes*		7-8
Brown bread	5-6	
Cooked chickpeas		5-10
Cooked lentils	4-5	
Dry dates		4-5
White bread		2-3
Whole rice		2-3
Orange*		2
Carrots*, leeks*	2-4	
Cabbage, spinach*, potatoes*	1-3	
Lettuces, fruits		1

* approximately 50% and more of soluble fibres

Many research studies had as an objective the study of the effect of dietary fibres on carbohydrate and lipid metabolism. This is because diabetes and cardiovascular diseases are at the forefront among pathologies in industrialised countries. Numerous experimental studies have shown that various sources of dietary fibre induce a significant decrease in post-prandial glycaemia and insulinemia. After chronic enrichment of diet, fasting glycaemia and insulin requirements can be decreased.

At the same time, many experimental studies carried out in animals and humans have shown that chronic addition of certain sources of dietary fibre to the diet (especially soluble viscous fibres) can favourably modify certain blood lipid parameters (cholesterolemia and LDL cholesterol). Epidemiological studies have shown a negative correlation between fibre ingestion and cardiovascular risk. A Mediterranean type diet, rich in fibre and low in saturated lipids, results in a decrease of 12-14% of cholesterolemia and LDL cholesterol in comparison with the current average diet.

For these reasons, it is advised to increase the portion of dietary fibre in the habitual diet, for example by rehabilitating the Mediterranean diet. Based on the result of epidemiological studies showing a decrease in relative risks above 25 g/day, the recommendations are to consume at least 25 g/day or even better 30 g/day of fibres.

Eating behaviour and culinary practices

Eating behaviour and culinary practices
Martine Padilla, Françoise Aubaille-Sallenave, Bénédicte Oberti

It seems more and more established that traditional Mediterranean diet responds to the preventative nutritional recommendations for the major endemics of our society. If this fact enters the social field of consumption attitudes, it could have major implications on public health (cardiovascular diseases are the major cause of mortality and morbidity in France with 20 000 deaths per year). Manufacturers, concerned with maintaining or creating a new market, have taken over the image to promote products. This marketing position is important for their strategic decisions in terms of products, brands, and markets (innovation, product management, communication).

This "nutritional culture" may be seen as a true society phenomenon, especially in English-speaking countries, while the identity of all the elements responsible for the health benefit have yet to be identified. This phenomenon if it takes place in a disorderly fashion and without any scientific basis, might lead to a break up and devaluation of this mode of eating, and reinforce its detractors.

Beyond the foods and nutrients that compose the Mediterranean diet, which seem to have an impact on health prevention (*see Part I*: "Epidemiology"), it appears also essential to contemplate the behaviour handed down throughout history, the transfers of people and cultural practices. It is indeed undeniable that the major constituents to be maintained must be identified, but is it not also an eating attitude or behaviour that must be acquired, found again, or preserved? In the United States and Great Britain, certain dietary recommendations have been well integrated into public health policies. The Mediterranean diet pyramid is well-placed in the US Department of Health and Human Services documents, and the ministries of health in England and Australia are largely inspired by it in their recommendation-prevention campaigns. Several surveys revealed that the principles have been well-understood and integrated by the population. A European survey (Zunft *et al.*, 1997) revealed the existence of a collective conscience of a healthy diet: according to the interviewees to stay in good health, prevent diseases, guarantee a quality of life and control weight gain, the following must be done in hierarchical order of importance: consume more fruits and vegetables, less fat, watch the ration balance, eat as much as possible fresh and natural products, few additives, less meat and sugar, and make sure to consume fibres. In spite of the incorporation of this knowledge, the modifications of eating behaviour expected did not follow (Hulshof *et al.*, 1993; DHHS, 1994). Therefore, little or no incidence on the regression of diseases and obesity can be observed. We can ask ourselves about the partial incorporation of all the recommendations, and especially if they have really taken into account the attitudes? Indeed, this can be partly attributed to the fact that most of the nutritional recommendation programmes have been developed based on epidemiological and socio-demographic data; they have failed at the application level due to their ignorance of eating behaviour and strategies that would help the populations to accept the change (Heimendiger and Van Duynm 1995). The most often cited barriers that prevent the adoption of the eating behaviours are the following: fast life style (lack of time), irregularity of working hours and giving up loved food (Kearney et al., 1997). Food industry innovation would thus have an important role to play in proposing natural, nutritional, practical and tasty foods.

Modernity destabilises the eater's references: loss of "true taste", fear of degradation of food quality, fear of eating in isolation. This results in a search for a strong identity. This re-appropriation of a traditional eating scheme would lessen the effects of the disappearance of society eating behaviour. But what are the traditional eating behaviours in the Mediterranean zone, what is special about their culinary practice? Finally, do we know if these practices have a relationship with health? This is what we will try to analyse in this chapter.

EATING BEHAVIOUR

Diversity

Diversity appears between countries, at the level of the entire Mediterranean zone and within each country, at the level of dietary rations.

An apparently homogenous region such as all the Mediterranean countries within the European Union, presents within itself noticeable differences, that reflect the methods of production *(figure 1)*. Spain and Portugal are characterised by a high consumption of potatoes, fish and seafood; Italy is mostly a cereal (the famous pasta) and milk consumer. In Greece the consumption leans mostly towards cereals, fruits, vegetables and feta. Unsurprisingly, France is undoubtedly the most "westernised" Mediterranean country with a high meat and dairy product consumption. Geographical proximity also plays a major role in the distribution of eating habits. Greece and Portugal that do not have a direct border with Northern Europe, keep a relatively traditional model. Also, it is true that apart from this relative natural protection, they have the lowest living standards in the European Union, which has not incited the major food industries and distributors (strong dietary change vectors) to massively invest in these countries. Food reflects the history of nations and does not respect geographical borders: Greece is strongly influenced by a more Oriental cuisine, Spain, like Sicily, is strongly marked by the Moorish past; French Provence resembles Italy a great deal (Padilla, 1996).

Numerous parameters have played a role in the diversity of foods and behaviours in Mediterranean regions.

– The geographical milieu, which is very heterogeneous and very contrasting, allows the cultivation of cereals, mixed crops, horticultural crops, perennial fruit tree cultivation, as well as bovine, ovine and goat breeding. Of course, sea fishing is present everywhere but remains coastal.

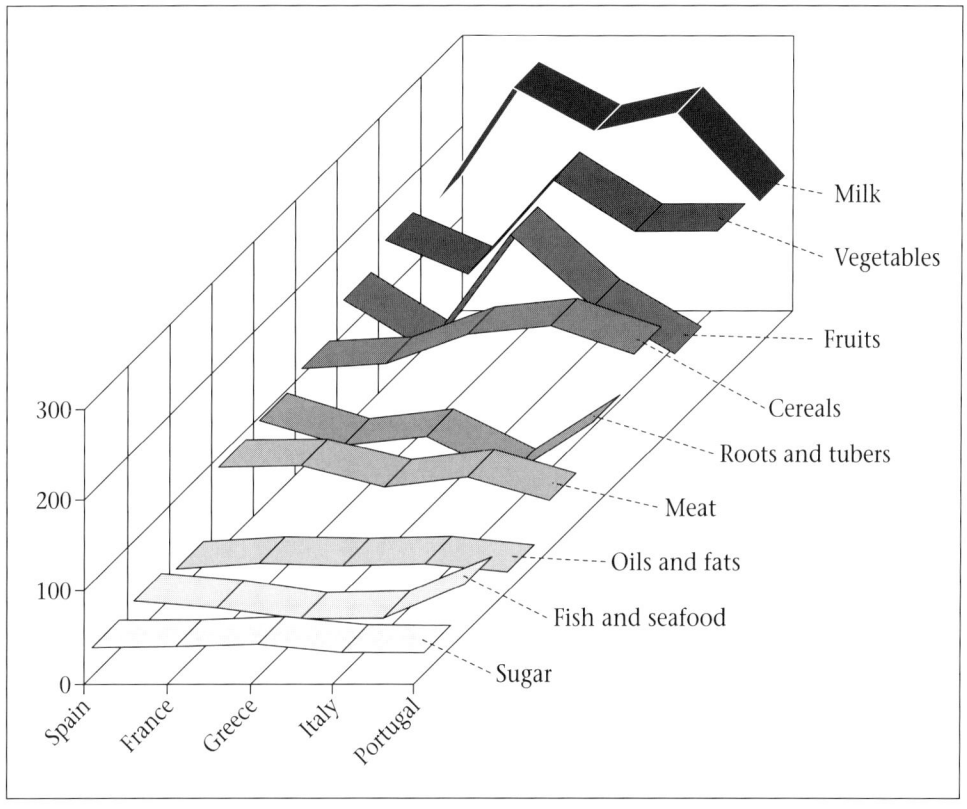

Figure 1. Examples of the diversity of food availability in the Mediterranean zone.

– Then with the appearance of new foods brought by each dominant population, the Greeks, Carthaginians and Romans, brought the vines, olive trees and fruits and vegetables from the Near East; Arabs, Byzantines and Ottomans brought numerous Oriental vegetables and culinary practices; Spanish and Portuguese did the same with American vegetables *(figure 2)*. With the contribution of new techniques: the Teutons taught the practice of soup making, the Muslims developed frying and also contributed to complex and refined preparations such as Persian pastries (Aubaile in Padilla 2000, Padilla *et al.*, 1998).

– The essential role played by cities and ports in the mixing of cultures and food should not be forgotten. The strong opposition between these sites of diversity and the countryside, more homogeneous, where diet is monotonous and often poor, should be noted.

As the exchanges of products and species are almost finished, this great diversity has come today to its maturity. A recent study has demonstrated this reality by comparing the diversity of the French diet with the American diet. A diversity indicator has been developed by the Food Consumption Observatory using the same methodology in France and in the United

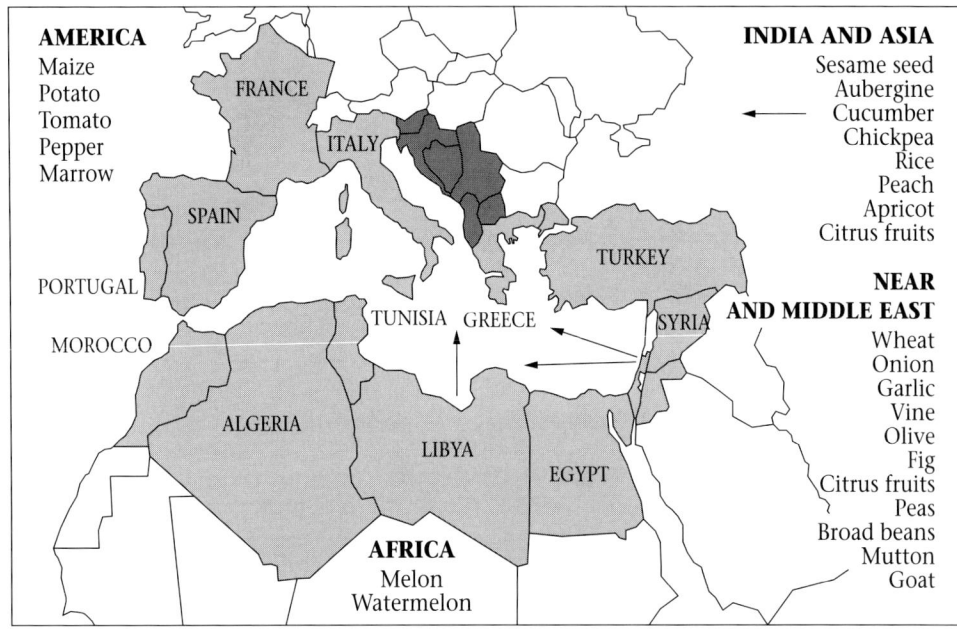

Figure 2.

States. Based on the number of different categories of foods consumed the same day, it shows the gap between the two continents: 56% of French consumers reach the maximum diversity level, only 34% of Americans are in that case (Volatier, 1999).

A pilot study of dietary behaviour in Europe provides us with interesting comparative information, especially in what concerns the diversity aspect[1]. England differs in this from the United States; it seems that its colonial past has greatly influenced the dietary repertory. A great variety of vegetables and cooking techniques are employed, herbs and spices are occasionally appreciated. Exotic dishes are in progression to the detriment of traditional English dishes. Their taste for sugar makes them appreciate Mediterranean desserts which often include honey. In other European countries, such as Belgium, consumption is relatively monotonous, without a marked seasonal influence. Culinary techniques are not very varied; they are mainly satisfied with soups and roasts (Gerber and Padilla, 1998).

---

1. This project "Consommer méditerranéen, une action préventive au cancer" was coordinated by Gerber M/INSERM/CRLC) and Padilla M (CIHEAM/IAMM) and associated Huber A (CNRS/University of Bordeaux), Hladik M (Museum of Natural History), Macbeth H (University of Oxford Brookes), Guillaume M (CNRN/Brussels), Gonzalez Turmo I (University of Seville), Fanfani R, Gatti S (University of Bologna), Cresta M (University of Rome).

This Mediterranean diversification was born under the very strong influence of the Hippocratic medical system[2]. This system considers that animal and vegetable products have hot or cold, and dry or wet properties. These properties are combined two by two to form the specific nature of each food. The ideal is to diversify and preserve a balance between the different natures of the products, as a function of the season, the nature and the condition of the consumer. This system, widely spread and popularised by medieval Jewish and Muslim physicians, remains today highly present in popular knowledge.

Acquisition behaviours

Food acquisition modes do not seem to present any particularity within the Mediterranean zone; they largely depend on the dissemination of distribution commercial spaces (presence or not of supermarkets or superstores), but also the local customs. In France in the Herault department, consumers buy their provisions in supermarkets or superstores, however the exchanges of pick-your-own or parental garden products are frequent. Freezing or "home-made preserves" remain common practice. In the Tarn, a very rural department, the poultry products reared by the parents are appreciated, as well as direct buying at the farmhouse. This applies to all foods: in town, fresh produce markets are visited when one cannot obtain these products from the family. In rural Italy, family production remains important, as well as direct sales from shepherds and farmers. However, in Spain, food is bought from shopkeepers, even in the countryside: very few vegetable gardens, no pick-your-own farms.

In Belgium while supermarket shopping is the general rule, the practice of pick-your-own is frequent and households often have their vegetable gardens. In England, numerous families cultivate aromatic herbs in their gardens (Gerber and Padilla, 1998).

A strong link to traditional peasant diet is seen from the analysis of habits and values. This link goes through the shopping methods characterised by home-production and going to the market. Certainly the weight of home-production in total consumption varies with age; very high among the elderly, it becomes less essential for the younger generations. We go from a production experienced as a necessity to a production experienced as a hobby. The practice of storage, yet again, reveals the weight of the traditional model, especially in the confection of domestic preserves (jams, vegetables, animal fats, etc.). These traditional practices are also found in the Southern and Eastern Mediterranean countries, for example with the *Mouné* in Lebanon (Kanafani, 1994).

Of course almost everywhere, at least in Europe, freezers are widely used and their large sizes reveal that the storage behaviour, which evolves as a function of technological transformations, remains rooted in the mentalities.

---

2. Medicine on which Western European medieval and classic medicines were based, thanks to the Syriac and then Arab and finally Latin translations of Greek works by this physician from the IVth century B.C.

Meal structures

Throughout the Mediterranean countries, lunch remains the main meal. However a swing towards the evening meal is observed, due to the organisation of the working day related to the instauration of continuous working days and the increasing distance between the work site and the home.

In France, lunch remains quantitatively more important. The evening meal is considerably simpler: it remains complete, that is comprising a starter, a main course, cheese and dessert in only 24% of cases (CREDOC, 1997).

However, the most socially significant meal is the evening meal: Today, 84% of families eat together in the evening; its duration is important: 33 minutes during the week, 43 minutes during the weekend. The increase in the duration of breakfast confirms the attachment to traditional meals: 18 minutes during the week, 22 during the weekend (Volatier, 1999).

"The simplicity of the meal structure in the North of France is better explained by ancient cultural differences than by a recent behaviour change in the younger generations" (Volatier, 1999). This meal permanence does not prevent the development of "between meal" eating, especially in young adults and adolescents, but they do not substitute the meals.

In Spain, the most important meal seems to be lunch; the evening meal is often lighter (salad, omelette). For the young, lunch is limited to sandwiches or pizzas. However, the organisation of work involves more and more, a consumption of lunch away from home, especially for men.

In the South of Italy, the traditional model is found both in the number of dishes presented (a single dish composed of pasta, vegetables and leguminous plants) as by the social aspect of the meal (presence of guests strangers to the family).

In Southern and Eastern Mediterranean people, "go home" for lunch whenever possible. Is the reason the attachment to traditions and the family or the lack of satisfactory collective eating structures?

In comparison, in Great Britain the main meal is breakfast. Furthermore, meals are highly unstructured and do not follow any rule for the sequence of the dishes; the English frequently practice "snacking", commonly use industrial preparations, pizzas, chips, etc. However a structuring effort is made for Sunday lunch often with the family.

In Belgium meals still seem to be structured, however with a swing of the main meal towards the evening meal, for reasons of family and work organisation. Whenever possible, lunch is eaten at home. It is considered as a "complete" meal because it compulsorily includes meat, vegetables, starches, etc.

Breakfast is very different in English-speaking countries and in Mediterranean countries (Grivetti, 1997). The English breakfast defined, in the last 1,000 years, as the three "B": beef, beer and bread, has evolved to a wide variety of dishes taken with tea or coffee. Historically, the English breakfast is rich and reflects the caloric and fat requirement for 12 to 15 hours of daily work in cold and humid weather conditions. It varies between 500 to 1,500 kcal. On the other hand, the Mediterranean breakfast is perceived as light: bread, biscuits and pastries dominate, accompanied by coffee and sometimes milk. It only contains 300 to 500 kcal. Just like beer was the morning drink in English-speaking countries, wine seemed to have the place of honour in Mediterranean countries, before the appearance of coffee and tea.

A wide diversity in breakfast content is observed in Mediterranean countries:

For example, in Greece in rural areas it includes bread, cheese, coffee and goat's milk, fruits and olives. In urban areas, to coffee and milk are added pastries, fruit juice, preserved fruits, eggs with ham and sausages, or cheese and butter. In Spain it only includes coffee and pastries *(churros)*; what differentiates individuals is the place where it is consumed: at home, at the café or at work. When taken at a café breakfast often starts with an aperitif, the *pacharron*. In rural Egypt, it is limited to coffee or tea sometimes accompanied by bread, onion and salt. In the urban zone of Cairo, the basic triad remains: coffee or tea, goat cheese and bread served with broad beans. Broad bean stew is sometimes accompanied by eggs or thin slices of smoked meat *(basturma)*. In Italy, it is limited to a cappuccino with wheat biscuits and sometimes a fruit, it remains very light: only 200 to 400 kcal (Toma, in Grivetti, 1997). In Turkey, breakfast is comprised of Turkish coffee or tea, cheese, raw vegetables and olives.

Conviviality

"The resistance of food to the North American model is stronger than that in the other domains such as television or cinema. This can be explained by the essential role of food in France and in Southern Europe as a conviviality vector and a means to strengthen social links" (Volatier, 1999). The studies of the CREDOC (1997) clearly showed that "getting together" was the first motivation of a meal eaten together, well before the quality of the food or the speed or the good development of the meal. The collective dimension of eating is essential because it reinforces solidarity and "living together" in everyday life that is often considered as stressful or functional.

The continuing interest in meals resides in the emergence of worries about food safety and a renewal in the interest for natural products. "This reassurance" favours little or not transformed products which are consumed during family meals. This strong tendency is not a simple fashion, it is favourable to regional products, and tends to unquestionably preserve a structured eating.

In France, the desire to express oneself through the preparation of meals is strong. It is true that the time dedicated to it decreases, but occasionally it can become a pleasure. The increasing participation of children and partners in the preparation of meals favours variety and the fun aspect of the elaboration of dishes: only 46% of men participated occasionally in the preparation of meals in 1988; they were 57% in 1997. The kitchen is increasingly a convivial room where everyone meets (CREDOC, 1997).

Eating outside is not a common practice in the Mediterranean countryside. Women do not show themselves much, especially in Muslim societies. However, religious and social feasts, and social visits are occasions to meet: the *nzhât* in the Maghreb are real parties of pleasure for the taste buds in the country or in a garden.

To meet around a drink, share a meal are necessary marks of conviviality and cohesion of a group. Inversely from women, men go out to meet in the café, under the shadow of a tree or in a village common room. Around a drink they eat in a relaxing atmosphere *petiscos* in

Portugal, *tapas* in Spain, *tramessi* in Italy, *kemya* in Tunisia, *meze* in Lebanon or *mezelik* in Turkey.

Changes in diet or habits

In the Mediterranean countries, unlike what is described currently in the Western world, women of all generations generally cook every day. However, the young adapt their mother's culinary practices simplifying the meals and including less fat and meat. The involvement in food is great. Knowledge can be passed between generations, and especially from mother to daughter. In France 41% of culinary specialities were transmitted in this way versus only 20% by cookery books.

However, eating behaviour rooted in a culinary culture is not static. On the contrary, the scope for innovation is wide.

In the Herault, the young generations cook like their parents: the girls follow the same recipes as their mothers, but making some changes, of which the main one is the decrease in the amount of lipids and sugars. In other words, they do the same recipes but in a lighter version; furthermore, they diversify their culinary repertory by introducing new dishes often of Mediterranean origin (couscous, paella, pizza, pasta). Women in the Tarn have not abandoned the ovens, and preserves as well as the freezing of seasonal produce are regularly carried out.

In Southern Italy, culinary discoveries are rare and the reticence about innovation has been shown to be strong. In Sicily, MacDonald's fast foods had to close due to lack of interest of the population.

In Spain, traditional food persists and a similarity of culinary practice between mothers and daughters is observed (except for olive oil which tends to be abandoned in cooking).

Four types of evolution can be noted, especially in the Northern Mediterranean zone.

– First there is a transformation of the representations concerning certain categories of food: the most prominent are cereals, with a transition from pasta towards rice and the regression of white bread replaced by whole or traditional wheat bread, a greater value given to sugar in festive meals, and a strong regression of cold cuts and cheeses.

– Then, there is the presence of children who influence the family choices (especially in Spain).

– Followed by the modification of women's status that has repercussions on the time spent in the kitchen. It results in a simplification of culinary practices (the rhythm of life requires a fast cooking), a preference for shopping in supermarkets (everything is in the same place) and a modification in the structure of meals (fewer sequences and more single dishes).

– Finally, the representations of the food/health link which evolve from cooking that "sticks to your ribs" to a lighter cuisine, symbolic of the dynamism which is supposed to represent the image of a svelte body. This transformation goes through a lipophobic attitude which results in a valorisation of fat poor food (vegetables, fruits, fish), but most of all by a loss of the central value given to meat that is observed in the younger generations (Padilla and Gerber, 1998).

Relationship to food

The discourse related to food is very variable depending on the country, even among Mediterranean countries: while England shows a great culinary curiosity, especially towards exotic dishes; Southern Spain still has a survival speech; perhaps the times of shortages and poverty are not sufficiently far behind? The hedonistic dimension is scarcely mentioned. On the other hand, France and Italy have a very detailed and varied culinary discourse with a strong hedonistic component. For the French to "eat" represents life (for 27%), pleasure (for 26%), and health (for 22%) (CFES, 1997).

Rural zones, indistinctly, do not construct reflections on their diet: rural families whether they are from the Tarn (France), Ronda (Spain) or Cilento (Italy) are incapable of describing the specificity of their culinary traditions, unlike the urban or neo-rural families which develop the pleasure and health aspect of a traditional diet.

CULINARY PRACTICES

The notion of Mediterranean diet comprises a very large number of different cuisines from which the common characteristics should be extracted. A study (Aubaille-Sallenave, 1996) was carried out as a reaction to the general statements of certain American and European dieticians who oversimplify and reduce the diet of Mediterranean peoples to a single model: that of Calabria emigrants in New York or that of the inhabitants of Crete or Southern Italy. Here is the broad outline.

Sobriety and frugality

These two characteristics of Mediterranean diet are mainly due to unfavourable economic conditions. Until the Second World War under-nourishment remained a frequent phenomenon throughout the Mediterranean zone, including the North. Currently, certain ideas prevail, abundantly disseminated by the media that advocate an ideal: a Mediterranean cuisine considered as unique, unchanging if not thousand of years old. This immediately conflicts with the question of the nature, unity or diversity of Mediterranean cuisine. Numerous questions come to mind: is there a Mediterranean cuisine? Does the cuisine of Seville resemble that of Marseilles or Beirut? Do Mediterraneans eat today what they used to eat in the past? Can it be said in the end whether this cuisine is a myth or a reality? The essence of a cuisine is based on the products used, as well as on the beliefs, know-how, food cooking methods and the way they are eaten.

Herbs

They occupy a prime place in dietetics, due to their hot properties, where both their prophylactic and curative action involves the appreciation of flavours. Thus thyme, sage, rosemary and almost all condiments find their place in popular dietetics. Aromatic herb infusions are commonly drunk for their digestive aide action. To qualify winter or summer foods seemed to be the expression of a well-being admitted by all. This concept is based on the humoral system which ruled learned medicine and whose goal was to make food as effective and digestible as possible, for each case, and whenever necessary to use their prophylactic or curative action, without forgetting the hedonistic dimension. Cuisines taking into account these medical parameters belonged to a learned culture, however a significant part of this knowledge passed into popular culture.

Culinary techniques

Mediterranean cuisine, due to the variety of preparation, cooking and preservation techniques and everything that comes into the preparation of a meal, is prepared in several steps and requires time. These are the peculiarities of these cuisines.

The diverse techniques are destined to make the food tastier and make them give the best of themselves.

As for the **preparation techniques**: the seasoning of meats and fish before cooking, breading for frying, finely chopped food for fast cooking and accentuation of flavours, introduction into a dough to make the products more digestible, stuffing, flaky pastry, larding or multiple salads.

As for **cooking techniques**: fast or slow, they must always cook food well. The variants are numerous:

– boiling to obtain a stock, soups or mash;

– simmering for stews and sauces;

– roasting or grilling for festive occasions;

– frying (this technique is omnipresent in its mild form as the base of all sauces and stews);

– more rarely, cooking in vine or cabbage leaves;

– finally, steaming, a technique especially used in Northern Africa.

As for **preservation techniques**: there is oven or sun drying, salting, fermentation, vinegar or oil preserves and conserves in fat. It should be noted that smoking is not a Mediterranean technique, but of Northern Europe, it was brought to Spain and Italy probably by the Celts, great lovers of smoked meats.

Composition of meals

The meal is generally composed of a basic food made up of carbohydrates to which is associated the qualitative element of the meal which forms the accompaniment. In the Mediterranean countries, the basic food is made up of cereals and/or leguminous plants: It is a distinctive cultural mark: schematically in Italy they are pasta, rice (which substituted beans in certain regions) and maize; in metropolitan France they are bread and potatoes, in Portugal, they are potatoes, rye and maize bread; in Northern Africa hard wheat and barley, in Egypt rice, wheat and broad beans; in Anatolia, maize.

Eating behaviour and culinary practices

Condiments and spices

They play a primordial role in these cuisines. Strong aromas and flavours play an often ambivalent role; they are both drugs and food.

The variety of condiments is abundant. Few can leave indifferent; we find garlic, onion, parsley, peppers, sage, bay, olives, mint, basil, fresh coriander, aniseed and many more. It should be noted that aniseed is one of the most valued flavours in pastries and alcoholic beverages. Cheese, wine or vinegar can also be used as condiments, especially in fatty meat dishes or heavy starches.

Spices are less present than condiments. The varieties, quantities and combinations used vary a great deal depending on the cuisine. We find saffron, cinnamon, cumin, whole coriander, clove, nutmeg or ginger.

Flavours

The favourite flavours in the Mediterranean are the following:

– acid: frequent use of vinegar, lemon and other citrus fruit juice to find this flavour;

– sweet and sour;

– sweet and salty: a flavour similar to sweet and sour, present in some sauces, meat and fish dishes as well as desserts;

– bitter: it has a dietetic and medicinal connotation for its heat and dryness, bitterness which is a fairly disagreeable flavour finds a positive value and even becomes strongly appreciated, especially in numerous aperitif drinks;

– hot: it is not a flavour, but it belongs to the tactile field and is felt when the trigeminal nerve is touched. It is found in garlic, pepper, sweet pepper, and hot pepper. Therefore, it belongs here.

Seasonality

Consumption is influenced by seasons. Indeed, in a climate where the contrast between seasons is marked by significant temperature differences, between 5 to 45° C, a balance between ambient temperature and body temperature should be established. Summer food should be refreshing by its cold properties: tomatoes, vinegar, lettuce, young meat, etc. On the contrary, winter food have hot properties: garlic, cabbage, fatty meat, etc. Thus vegetables and meats have always been in keeping with the seasons.

The contrast is also noted in the preparations: winter dishes and summer dishes. The gazpachos, sort of cold soup from Southern Spain, are hot in winter, The contrast also exists in the drinks: between the winter sugared and spiced winter infusions and the acid fruit, flower juices or buttermilk based drinks *(leben, labneh)*.

In spite of the diversity of regions, relief, religions, languages, we can talk of Mediterranean cuisines or actually cuisines, the plural being used for multiple recipes and the singular encompassing everything they have in common. This community expresses itself in multiple techniques, competences and modes of preparations, but also in dietetic knowledge and beliefs. There is a great curiosity for subtle flavours and tastes. All these factors facilitate the borrowing, allow adaptation to new products and open up to the creation of new recipes.

Everything shows that the Mediterranean, in spite an often forced sobriety, knows how to appreciate both the variety of flavours as that of odour and colours.

Aesthetics is a major component of these cuisines, a visual aesthetic with the mixing of colours.

Each of these traits, each of these techniques, each of these products are certainly not exclusive or specific to Mediterranean cuisines; they can all be found in other cuisines. However, the fact of finding them together, combining them and creating a harmony is what makes up the specific characteristic of Mediterranean cuisines.

LINKS BETWEEN DIETARY HABITS AND HEALTH

According to Salen and De Lorgeril (1997), the apparently natural protection of Mediterraneans is not hereditary; when Mediterraneans emigrate and adopt the lifestyle and dietary habits of the host countries, they are rapidly subjected to the high risks of infarction. The link between the dominant elements of their diet (variety) and also the dietary habits (structure of meals, conviviality) seem to be involved.

Variety

Willet *et al.* (1995) believe that Mediterranean diet provides all micronutrients and fibres due to its **variety**. Industrial transformation is minimal, seasonality is respected, products are brought and prepared fresh, which preserves a maximum of micronutrients, antioxidants and minimises harmful substances. This leads to wonder about industrial products. Does their mode of production destroy these life substances or does it bring allergenic or harmful substances? One can only recommend to manufacturers to try to preserve micronutrients, vitamins and trace elements during the product transformation operations, and to limit the use of additives and other products likely to denature the foods.

Food intake

Is the fact of privileging breakfast beneficial? There is a nutritionist physicians "school" that believes that a light consumption after 5 p.m. is beneficial on a physiological level and limits obesity (Danguir and El Ati, 1995).

A comparative study between the United States and France was carried out in the beginning of the 1990s (Andersson-Hassam and Astier-Dumas, 1992) on the distribution of food intake throughout the day. The questioned subjects were asked to note their food intakes in order to try to determine if chronobiology phenomena could explain the differences of food physiological effects observed.

The average number of food intakes is not very different: 4 in France, 6 in the United States. However, the distribution of the energy consumption during the day is significantly different *(figure 3)*. In France, a small peak corresponding to breakfast is seen, then nothing until lunch which is the main meal. During the afternoon, consumptions are low or nil, then a new peak indicates dinner between 7 and 9 p.m. The American rhythm is very different, with a multiplication of small consumptions during the day.

When the distribution of the ingestions according to the major periods of the day, before or after 2 p.m. are analysed, it can be seen that most of the energy consumption (60%) is done before 2 p.m. in France, the opposite is true in the United States.

These results should be further examined to determine their significance on a metabolic level.

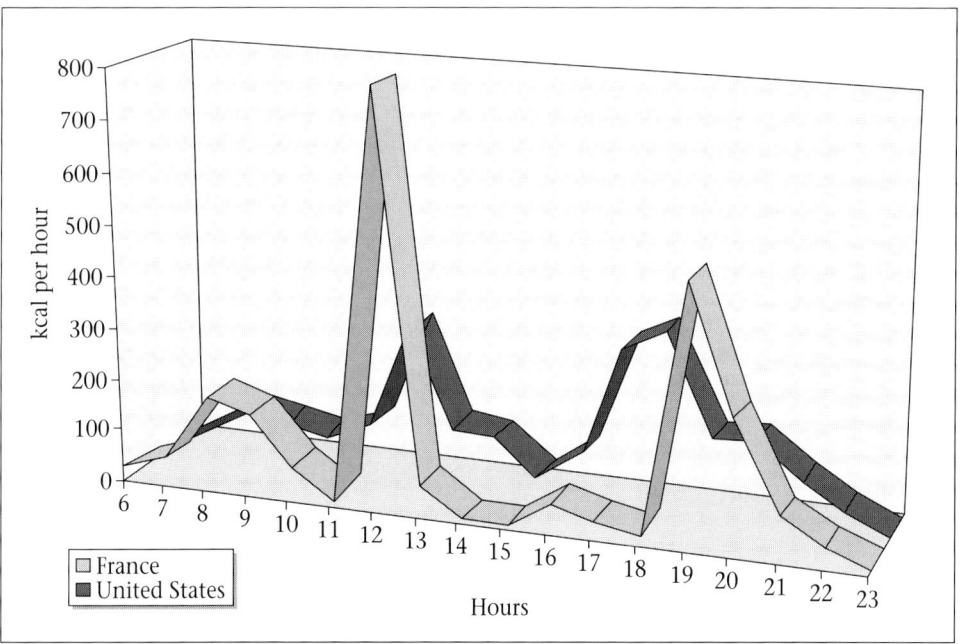

Figure 3. Daily distribution of energy intake. Source : Médecine et nutrition, 1992.

Lifestyle and conviviality

The **Mediterranean lifestyle** is particularly interesting: a sense of community (family, friends) is observed, meals are long and relaxing, varied dishes stimulate appetite by their colours, odours and flavours.

The Mediterranean lesson is not so much from the products, taken individually, that make it up but rather from the combination of food, of a way of eating and a variety of dishes. It is difficult, if not absurd, to want to transfer Mediterranean food in all its components, however it is possible to transmit a way of eating or a "dietary culture".

The Mediterranean lifestyle certainly contributes to a lower incidence in cardiovascular diseases: long and convivial meals release daily stress, the colours and flavours of dishes stimulate appetite, the practice of the siesta provides rest, relaxation and regeneration, the mildness of the climate encourages outdoor physical activities and extended families help social insertion (Willet *et al.*, 1995).

Finally, the basic lesson that can be extracted from this presentation of Mediterranean diet is that "eating well" is restored by "living well". Food and related practices are an essential component of health and the quality of life. The variety, organised and not anarchic, of dishes, culinary preparations, the respect of the seasons and the biological rhythm of humans, the sharing of the pleasures of the table are undoubtedly all keys to the "health effect" of Mediterranean diet. Its rediscovery requires measures with respect to the nutritional education of populations and especially the young, as well as an adaptation to a modern lifestyle to offer services and practical products to the consumer. Food technology can make a significant contribution in this point.

References

- Andersson-Hassam E, Astier-Dumas M. Le paradoxe français à la recherche d'une explication. *Médecine et Nutrition* 1992 ; 28(4) : 231-3.

- Aubaile-Sallenave F. La Méditerranée, une cuisine, des cuisines. Informations sur les sciences sociales, anthropologie de l'alimentation. *SAGE* 1996 ; 35(1) : 135-94.

- Avalonne MH. Qu'est-ce qu'on mange ce soir ? Contribution socio-anthropologique à une étude d'épidémiologie nutritionnelle. 1998.

- Braudel F. *La Méditerranée, l'espace et l'histoire*. Paris : Flammarion, 1985.

- Craik E. Hippokratic diaita. In : Wilkins J, Harvey D, Dobson M, eds., *Food in antiquity*. Univ. of Exeter Press, 1995 : 343-58.

- Danguir J, El Ati J. Free-day eating versus striet night-fasting induce long-term weight loss without calorie restriction in obese patients. The 6th European Congress on Obesity, Copenhagen, May 31-June 3, 1995.

- Ferro-Luzzi A, Branca F. Mediterranean diet, italian-style : prototype of a healthy diet. *Am J Clin Nutr* 1995 : 61 (Suppl.) : 1338S-45S.

- Fidanza A, Simonetti MS, Genipi L. The child of today and tne mediterranean diet. *Beitr Infusionsther*. Basel : Karger, 1991 ; vol. 27 : 152-60.

- Fitzpatrick J. An historical geography of mediterranean cuisines. *Westerly* 1994 ; 4 : 37-47.

- Gerber M, Padilla M. Consommer méditerranéen, une action préventive au cancer ; rapport CE DGV, Programme « Europe contre le cancer », décembre 1998.

- Grivetti L. Morning meals. North american and mediterranean breakfast patterns. *Nutrition Today* 1997 ; 32(4) : 164-71.

- Haber B. The mediteranean diet : a view from history. *Am J Clin Nutr* 1997 ; 66 (Suppl.) : 1053S-7S.

- Heimendinger J, Van Duyn M. Dietary behaviour change : the challenge of recasting the role of fruit and vegetables in the American diet. *Am J Clin Nutr* 1995 ; 61 (Suppl.) : 13875-4015.

- Hubert A. *Pourquoi les eskimos n'ont pas de cholestérol*. Paris : J'ai Lu, 1995.

- Hulshof K, Lowik M, Kistemaker C, Hermus RJ, *et al.* Comparison of dietary intake with guidelines, some potential pitfalls ; Dutch nutrition surveillance system. *J Am Coll Nutr* 1993 ; 12 : 176-85.

- Jenkins NH. *The mediterranean diet cookbook : a delicious alternative for lifelong health.* New-York : Bantam, 1994.

- Kanafani-Zahar A. *Mune : la conservation alimentaire traditionnelle au Liban.* Paris : Éditions de la Maison des sciences de l'homme, 1994, 262 p.

- Kearney JM, Kearney M, Gibney MJ. *European Journal of Clinical Nutrition* 1997 ; 51 (Suppl. 2) : S57-S58.

- Maff. *The dietary and nutritional survey of British adults.* London : HMSO, 1994.

- Malassis L. *Nourrir les hommes.* Flammarion, 1994.

- Margetts BM, Martinez JA, Saba A, Holm L, Kearney M. Definitions of healthy eating : a pan-EU survey of consumer attitudes to food, nutrition and health. *Eur J Clin Nutr* 1997 ; 51 (Suppl. 2) : S23-S29.

- Mintz S. Eating and beeing, what food means. In : Harris-White B, Hoffenberg R, eds. *Food multidiciplinarity perspectives.* Oxford : Blackwell, 1994 : 102-15.

- Padilla M. L'alimentation méditerranéenne : une nouvelle référence internationale. *Cahiers de Nutrition et de Diététique* 1996 ; 4 : 204-8.

- Padilla M. L'alimentation méditerranéenne, une et plurielle. In : Padilla M, ed. *Aliments et nourriture sur le pourtour méditerranéen.* Paris : Karthala, 2000.

- Padilla M, Malassis L, Allaya M. *Que mangeons-nous ?* Agropolis Museum/CIHEAM-IAM, 1998.

- Padilla M, Gerber M. *Le consommateur face à l'alimentation méditerranéenne.* Rapport Conseil Régional Languedoc-Roussillon/CIHEAM-IAM, 1998.

- Sauner-Nebioglu MH. *Évolution des pratiques alimentaires en Anatolie : analyse comparative.* Berlin : Klaus Schwarz Verlag, 1995a.

- Sauner-Nebioglu MH. La cuisine turque. In : *Cuisines d'Orient et d'ailleurs.* Glénat, 1995b : 90-102.

- Trichopoulou A, Lagiou P. Healthy, traditional mediterranean diet : an expression of culture, history and life style. *Nutrition Rev* 1997 ; 55 : 383-9.

- US Department of Health and Human Services. Healthy people 2,000 : national health promotion and disease prevention objectives. US Government Printing Office, DHHS publication, 1990.

- Volatier JL. *Le repas traditionnel se porte encore bien.* CREDOC, Consommation et modes de vie, n° 132, 1999.

- Willett W, Sacks F, Trichopoulou A, Drescher G, Ferro-Luzzi A, Helsing E, Trichopoulos D. Mediterranean diet pyramid : a cultural model for healthy eating. *Am J Clin Nutr* 1995 ; 61 : 1402S-1406S.

- Wolfert P. *The cooking of the Eastern Mediterranean : 215 healthy, vibrant and inspired recipes.* New York : HarperCollins, 1994.

- Zunft HJ, Friebe D, Seppelt B, De Graaf C, *et al. Eur J Clin Nutr* 1997 ; 51 (Suppl. 2) : S41-S46.

Prospects for Mediterranean food

Preserve the health capital of food with appropriate technological treatments

Pierre Besançon

Any food must meet the double quality requirement of safety and acceptability *(figure 1)*; with priority being given to the guarantee of total harmlessness:

– on a microbiological level on the one hand (absence of pathogenic micro-organisms),

– and on a toxicological level on the other hand: absence of hazardous xenobiotics and the use of authorised additives and processing aids only.

Nutritional value is a function of the composition of different nutrients (amino acids, fatty acids, vitamins, mineral elements, fibres) as well as various micro-constituents which do not necessarily have a status of nutrient, but which play a beneficial protection role (anti-oxidants). Another very important component of nutritional quality is based on the notion of bioavailability of the various nutrients, i.e. their capacity of actually being released during the digestive processes, and to be correctly absorbed then efficiently used at a metabolic level. Therefore, the bioavailability of nutrients depends on their physico-chemical nature, their environment, on the presence of anti-nutritional factors, technological treatments or even the dietary balance and food rhythm.

The acceptability of food includes all the organoleptic qualities: flavours, aromas, colours, textures, etc. as well as the service qualities incorporated or combined with the commercialised product: for example, this is the case of ready to use food. All sorts of treatments, whether home, small scale or industrial, are essential for the elaboration of authentic food from agricultural raw materials which are not necessarily edible in nature, while conciliating safety and pleasure. The challenge is to preserve all the health capital of food by a judicious selection of appropriate and optimised technological processes.

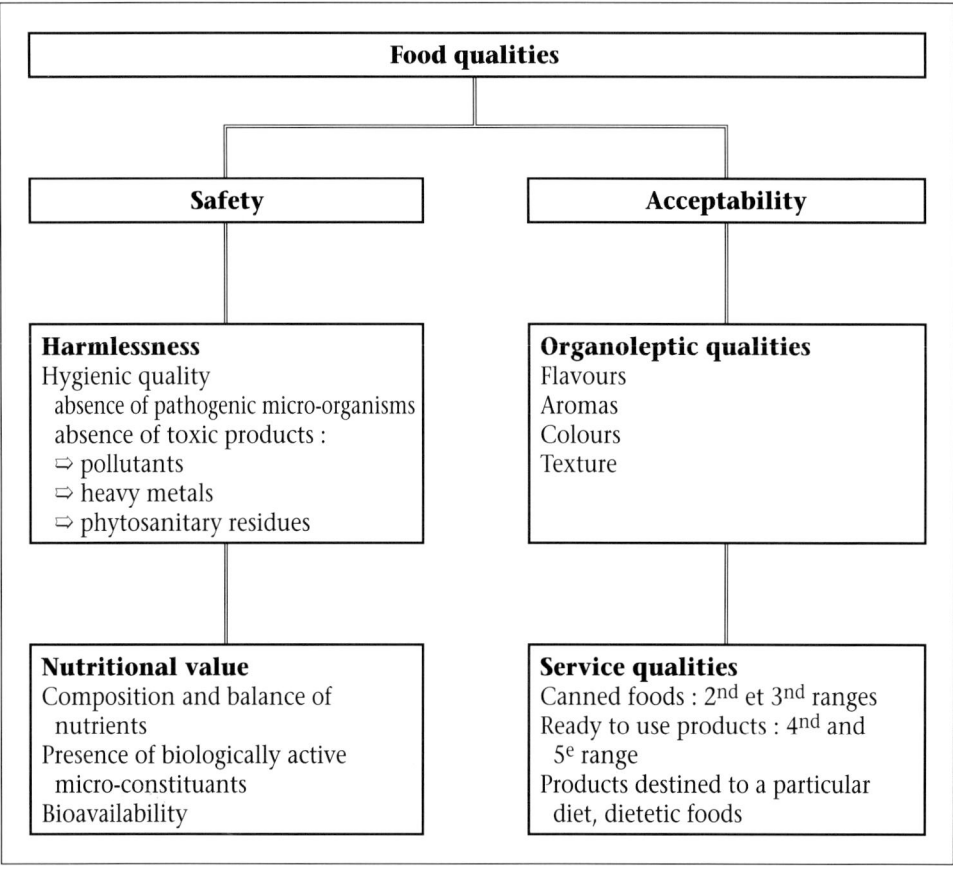

Figure 1. The double safety and acceptability requirement that guarantees the quality of any food.

TECHNOLOGICAL TREATMENTS

The different types of treatments used in the food industry have very varied objectives:

– separate, extract edible parts of plant or animal raw materials: husking, dressing, elimination of undesirable fat, etc.;

– refine or purify raw products: refining of oils, sugars, cereals, skimming of milk, etc.;

– allow and improve storage and preservation conditions by eliminating any risk of development of undesirable or pathogenic micro-organisms. Thermal (pasteurisation, sterilisation, freezing, deep-freezing) or biological (fermentation, enzymatic treatments) treatments are generally used. Other treatments also aim at limiting the activity of water: drying, pickling, preserving in sugar, osmotic dehydration. Finally, controlled atmospheres can be used to regulate metabolic paths (maturation, ripening) in the products being stored;

– modify and improve the functional or rheological properties of products: solubility, viscosity, fluidity, gel formation capacity, etc.;

– improve the organoleptic components or generate new sensory qualities: development of aromas, flavours by cooking, by fermentations, etc.;

– improve nutritional qualities by eliminating factors that play an anti-nutritional role on the bioavailability of nutrients (phytates, digestive enzyme inhibitors, excess fibres, etc.) by nutrient enrichment (supplementation, distillation, genetic engineering), by the preservation of non nutritional micro-constituents that play a protective role.

These objectives can be reached by the use of numerous physico-chemical or biotechnological processes, of which we can cite a few examples without being exhaustive.

- The physical processes include the following:
- thermal treatments by heat transfer: heating, pasteurisation, sterilisation, refrigeration, freezing, deep-freezing;
- mechanical treatments: grinding, centrifugation, filtration, high pressure;
- electromagnetic treatments: microwaves, pulsed electric fields, pulsed magnetic fields;
- irradiation treatments: X rays, gamma rays;
- molecular distillation treatments.

- The chemical processes comprise the following:
- alkaline treatments to detoxify or for the solubilisation and extraction of proteins;
- acid treatments for hydrolysis;
- oxidant treatments to detoxify or lower microbial load;
- reducing treatments to hydrogenate fats and modify molecular structures;
- treatments of addition or binding of chemical functional groups on food macromolecules (acylation);
- the use of gas and controlled atmospheres:
- texturing treatments for the creation of protective films.

- Under the biotechnological heading the following can be cited:
- enzymatic treatments to texture and modify macromolecular structures in order to improve functional properties (transesterification of triglycerides, texturing of proteins and carbohydrates), or to inactivate toxic compounds;
- fermentations that result in a series of traditional products (cheese, bread products, wine, beer, vinegar, etc.) or new products (metabolites, aroma precursors):
- genetic engineering which aims at improving the nutrient composition of genetically modified products (enrichment in certain amino acids, fatty acids, vitamins, etc.).

These examples merit to be developed but this is beyond the scope of this work.

EFFECTS OF TECHNOLOGICAL TREATMENTS ON NUTRITIONAL QUALITY

Due to their diversity and especially to the more or less severe treatment conditions, the nutritional effects vary *(figure 2)* and can be classified in three levels:

– favourable effects, if the treatment conditions are mild and well-controlled;

– a small loss in nutritional value, without toxicological consequence when the treatments are moderate;

– severe loss in nutritional value accompanied by the appearance of newly formed toxic compounds, in the most severe treatment conditions.

Favourable effects

The aim of some treatments can be the improvement of the nutritional quality of products which are not edible in their natural status; this is the case of cooking or blanching. As far as only the general conformation of macromolecules is modified, without alteration of constitutive molecules (primary structure of amino acids or fatty acids), an improvement in digestibility may be observed due to the thermal denaturing of the proteins, the gelatinisation of starch, inactivation of undesirable enzymes (lipoxygenases) and destruction of thermolabile anti-nutritional factors (protease inhibitors, leguminous plant lectins). Also, fermentation processes often improve the nutritional value of the substrate product (enrichment in certain vitamins, amino acids etc.).

Unfavourable effects

Numerous nutrient losses or reduction of bioavailability can be envisaged. First there is a loss in nutrients, often minerals, vitamins and sometimes proteins, *via* the elimination of unconsumed plant parts or animal tissues. The skimming of milk leads to a loss of lipid soluble vitamins (vitamin A and D), cereal refining eliminates most of the mineral and vitamin elements contained in the peripheral layers; even though it should be said that they are combined with factors that reduce their bioavailability (phytates and fibres); the aleuronic layer of cereal-grain, eliminated with the bran, contains proteins with a better amino acid balance than proteins found in the albumen. Rice steaming allows a migration in the centripetal sense of water soluble nutrients (vitamins, minerals, phenolic compounds) which leads to an enrichment of the grain after treatment. Finally, the refining of oils leads to the loss of phenolic compounds, carotenoids and vitamin E.

Losses can also take place by solubilisation and diffusion. The removal of low molecular weight molecules in the wash and/or cooking water is unavoidable. These losses can be limited by optimising the process (size of particles, amount of water, duration, temperature, pH, etc.).

Oxidation is a major cause of the degradation in nutritional quality. Vitamins, (carotenoids, tocopherols, vitamin C, folates), amino acids (methionine, cysteine), fatty acids (poly-unsaturated fatty acids) can be oxidised. The oxidation of vitamins can be catalysed by the

Preserve the health capital of food with appropriate technological treatments

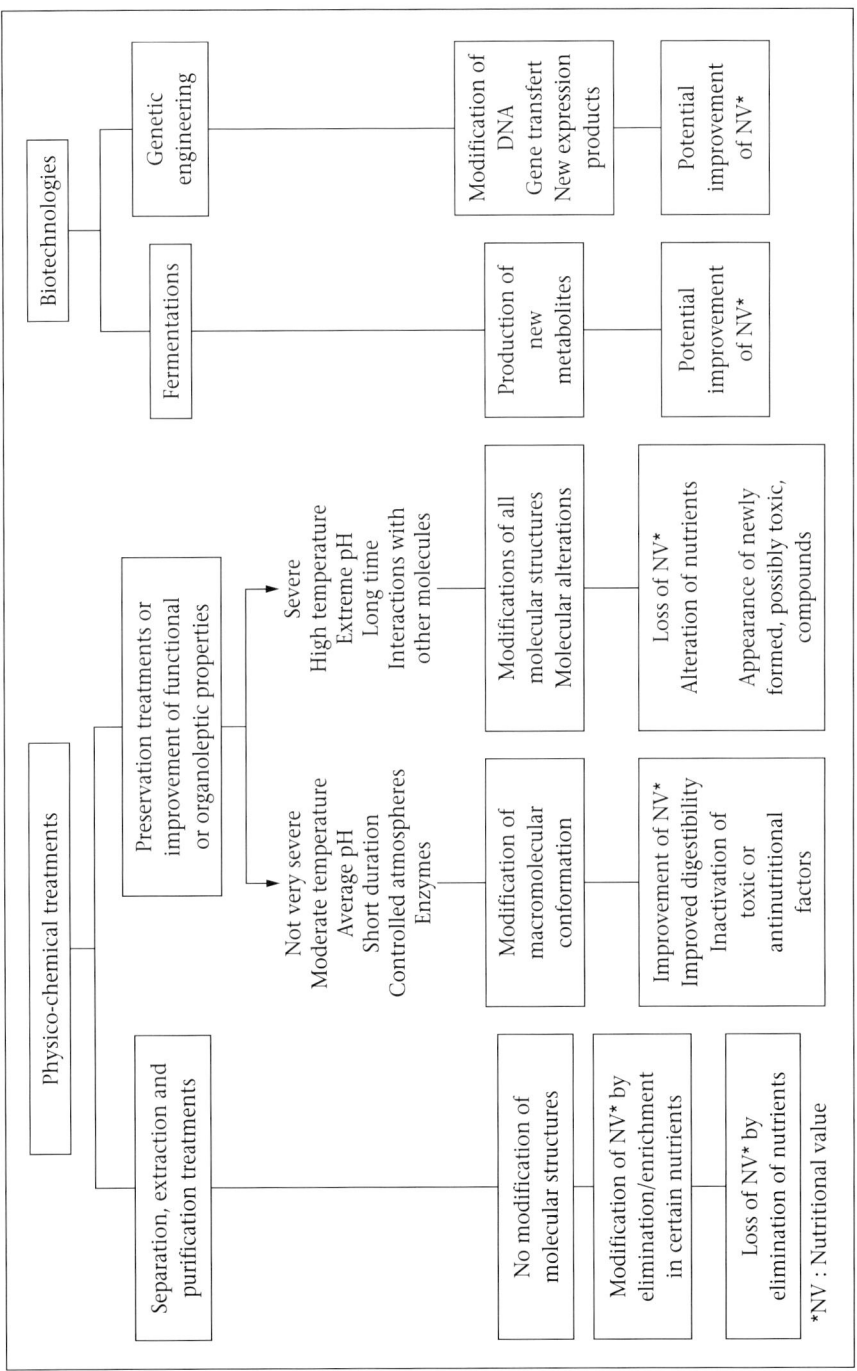

Figure 2. General effects of technological and biotechnological treatments on the nutritional value of food.

presence of metals (iron, copper), enzymes (oxydases) and accelerated by heat; it takes place during steam blanching and dehydration of vegetables (vitamin C), pasteurisation of milk (folates), frying (vitamin A and E). Vitamin losses take place throughout storage of food products and can be slowed down if the product contains anti-oxidant protection agents (presence of phenolic compounds) and if stored away from oxygen, under controlled atmosphere. Heat is always a deterioration factor for vitamin B1 and vitamin C, independently of oxidation effects.

It should also be mentioned that numerous compounds and additives can react with nutrients; sulphites deteriorate vitamin B1 and stabilise vitamin C, nitrates react with many vitamins, protein sulphydril groups (cysteine) with vitamins B6 and B12.

There are also many numerous causes of deterioration for amino acids (deamination, decarboxylation, isomerisation) under severe treatment conditions; addition and polymerisation compounds (Maillard's reaction in the presence of reducing sugars accelerated by thermic treatments) can appear as well as the formation of intramolecular covalent bonds (severe thermic and alkaline treatments). It is out of the question to mention here the possibility of forming toxic or mutagenic compounds under the most severe conditions. We will simply mention that the grilling of meat leads to protein and lipid deterioration products which are toxic and mutagenic.

Conclusion and prospects

Three objectives must be reached, and they are not totally compatible: food health safety, nutritional quality and sensory properties.

Insofar as the food network becomes more and more industrialised and collective eating develops, real compromises are required.

The first strategy consists in optimising treatments so as to guarantee maximum safety, which remains a priority, keep reasonable sensory qualities while maintaining a good nutritional quality. Sometimes smallest common denominator solutions are reached: choosing a sterilisation scale so as not to lose too many vitamins, not purify too much in order to avoid the risk of losing beneficial compounds (anti-oxidants) and other less interesting compounds.

The solution consisting in the extraction and purification of compounds considered as beneficial and their use as drugs is not necessarily the most interesting; it is beyond the scope of diet. The analysis of results of studies on the beneficial roles of certain foods or their constituents shows that synergic effects are as important as the sum of individual effects; this applies to natural anti-oxidants as it is more judicious to keep them in their food matrix.

Another approach is to implement new more selective processes with respect to the microbial flora, more respectful of cellular and molecular structures (polyphenols, carotenoids). The processes to be developed should also valorise the anti-oxidant potential of plants, as well as their enzymatic potential. Plant extracts (anti-oxidants, enzymes) may also offer interesting alternatives to the use of some additives and processing aids, without falling into the trap of thinking that everything that is natural is without danger!

Preserve the health capital of food with appropriate technological treatments

Industrial food technology is certainly not a necessary evil to create modern food, but should be rather considered as a useful partner, for the hygienist and nutrionist who wish to preserve or even develop the health capital of food.

REFERENCES

- Bernard A, Carlier H. Aspects nutritionnels des constituants des aliments. Influence des technologies. *Les Cahiers de l'ENSBANA*. Paris : Tec Doc, 1992, 392 p.

- Cheftel JC, Cheftel H, Besançon P. *Introduction à la biochimie et à la technologie des aliments*. Paris : Lavoisier, 1997, vol. 1, 381 p., vol. 2, 410 p.

- Cheftel JC, Cuq JL, Lorient D. *Protéines alimentaires*. Paris : Tec Doc., 1985, 308 p.

- Linden G, Lorient D. *Biochimie agroindustrielle*. Paris : Masson, 1994.

- Spinnler HE. Technologies de transformation des produits agroalimentaires. In : Baert JP, ed. *Agroalimentaire F1-170-1-14*. Paris : Techniques de l'Ingénieur, 1999.

- Tirilly A, Bourgeois CM. *Technologies des légumes*. Paris : Tec Doc., 1999, 558 p.

New agricultural practices and agro-food innovation to develop the health value of Mediterranean food

Stéphane Debosque, Marc Puygrenier

How to define a quality diet

In the previous chapters we have seen that to understand the nutritional "mechanisms" that play a role in keeping an individual or a population in good health, it is necessary to closely study the role of certain food constituents and micro-constituents. This is the usual operating procedure in scientific research, in all experimental science and life science fields.

However, we have also observed that the Mediterranean diet cannot be reduced to the sum of nutrients provided in a meal. Therefore, the evaluation of the quality of this diet must be carried out to optimise it in the future if possible.

Humans do not consume isolated foods separately, but combine them as a function of dietary habits. With respect to the Mediterranean diet, according to the established observations of epidemiologists and food behaviour specialists (*see Part I*: "Epidemiology"), these habits are healthy. For this reason instead of fixing amounts of each nutrient, nutritional recommendations should take the time to define a healthy, balanced diet and propose methods to determine the "overall" quality of the diet as a whole.

This is what proposes the so called "food pyramid-guide", issued from the work of the USDA (United States Department of Agriculture) which recommends a suitable balance between food groups (*see chapter* "Preserve and promote Mediterranean food for health: towards integrated nutritional policies").

The food groups to be consumed, recommended at a certain frequency, defined for the Mediterranean model (and more generally western) are the following:

– 1st group: cereals and starches (base of the pyramid), fruits and vegetables, olive oil and fresh cheeses or yoghurts which must be consumed daily;

– 2nd group: fish, poultry, eggs, sweets, accompanied of wine (1 or 2 glasses per day with meals) a few times a week;

– 3rd group: red meat, a few times a month (or a few times a week, in small quantities).

This "pyramid" is not the only one to be proposed. Other balanced diets have been defined for the same reasons as the "Mediterranean pyramid", thus a "Chinese" and a "British" pyramid have been mentioned. In all cases, a good balance can be measured by the food diversity score (FDS). It evaluates daily food consumption from the principal groups: cereals and starches, fruits and vegetables, dairy products and meat (for the Mediterranean model, *see the chapters* "Eating behaviour and culinary practices" and "Preserve and promote Mediterranean food for health").

Another evaluation criteria for the quality of a diet should be taken into account: moderation, especially with respect to lipid rich food and in particular in saturated fats, cholesterol, sugar and salt. The diet quality index (DQI) includes the observation of the moderation. In the Mediterranean model, olive oil is privileged and butter, red meat and dairy products are avoided.

Finally the food variety score (FVS), defined as " the number of different foods consumed during a given period of time", signals the dietary habits and the propensity to eat new foods relative to the previous days. All these criteria allow the evaluation of the overall healthy food index (OHFI) (cf. "Mediterranean pyramid" *see chapter* "Preserve and promote Mediterranean food for health").

Hedonism and conviviality could be added to this as has already been suggested in the "Eating behaviour and culinary practices" chapter. The taste of food and the pleasure derived from their consumption are a direct reflection of the quality of the diet (Drewnowski, 1999).

Thus, the Mediterranean diet cannot be disassociated from the life style in which it emerged, nor of the agricultural, rearing, fishing and fish farming products, the fruit of the work of men, of his experience and knowledge, but also of the climate and the exceptional amount of sunshine.

NEW AGRICULTURAL PRACTICES

"The essence of cooking (method of the preparation of food) is based, in agreement with Padilla and Aubaile-Sallenave (*see chapter* "Eating behaviour and culinary practices"), on the products used...". We will try to understand, by following the Mediterranean food "pyramid-guide", how agronomical research and the agricultural professions contribute to the development of the health value of products.

Cereals and starchy foods

While cereals are consumed in multiple forms at all meals for their carbohydrate content (starch), dietary fibres (whole cereals) also provide vitamins from the B group and proteins which are of interest because of their amino acid composition (*see chapter* "Beneficial effects of fruits and vegetables on health").

However, there are some, quite rare, cases of gluten intolerance. In young children and elderly persons, the phytate rich cereals can induce irritations of the digestive tube and mineral deficiencies (Champ, 1997).

The efforts of research and of the professionals are always made on the control of the quality of varieties, the sanitary quality (elimination of pesticides residues), the improvement and control of protein content for its consequences on technological aptitude and nutritional value. Indeed, nitrogen fertilisation remains not well enough elucidated to ensure a high quality protein content. Furthermore, varietal improvement, using the achievements of biotechnology within the context of a European project (PROTALL), aims to create wheat varieties that can be consumed by persons allergic to gluten (celiac disease). Employing the same genetic techniques, various works aim at developing the expression of wheat protein in order to improve their technological aptitude, for the manufacture of pasta ("behaviour" of pasta) and thermal stability of starch (amylose and amilopectin). Starch content was also increased in potatoes by the transfer of a gene to improve industrial use (for example mashed potatoes, potato starch, chips that absorb less frying oil) (*Les plantes génétiquement modifiées, une clef pour l'avenir*, 1997).

Fruits and vegetables

Fruits, vegetables and leguminous plants, advised daily in large amounts, have a protective effect against cardiovascular disease and cancers, especially of the digestive and upper respiratory-digestive tracts, stomach, lung, bronchi, pancreas, cervix and bladder, according to the reviews presented (see chapter "Health benefits of the Mediterranean consumption model). Most epidemiological studies consider the nutrients contained in these foods: fibres, water-soluble vitamins, anti-oxidants, folates and minerals.

These seasonal products, often consumed fresh in the summer production period, are highly diversified. They are preserved according to modern techniques (freezing) or traditional practices (drying, salting, vinegar or oil preserves, etc.) (*see chapter* "Eating behaviour and culinary practices").

The research-development efforts in this field were based on alternative methods to fight against the risk of presence of insecticides residues. Thus, research concentrates on the control of major diseases of fruit trees (chlorotic leafroll of apricot trees, pox common to apricot, peach, plum and cherry trees). At the same time, experiments are carried out on the evaluation of the sensitivity of stocks (Labonne *et al.*, 1999, Quiot *et al.*, 1999).

Overall, on a technical level the objective is the absence of pesticide residues and nitrates, the lengthening of the duration of production, especially by developing covered production.

Furthermore, research-development with lettuce producers as for most market gardening, aims at improving competitiveness and quality, by developing varietal choice, the type of cover adapted to an increased productivity, a conduct of tensiometry assisted irrigation according to "lettuce quality" specifications, as well as the choice of tools for working the soil (Peyrière *et al.*, 1999).

Finally, as for the fruits, alternative and biological control of parasite (thrips and aleurodes) programmes of vegetable farming allow the improvement of quality and food safety.

On a longer term, the search for new varieties or the modification of varieties for certain characteristics or capacities are the subject of work that aims at improving their quality. Thus, for lettuces or spinach, it is envisaged to reduce the nitrate content in leaves by increasing the expression of an enzyme that degrades nitrates (nitrate-reductase).

Research carried out with potato, tomato, cucumber, melon, pumpkin and beetroot will attempt at introducing a specific gene that will allow these plants to make a protein that stops the multiplication and development of pathogenic viruses (*Les plantes génétiquement modifiées, une clef pour l'avenir*, 1997).

Also, work is being carried out on the stimulation of resistance of radishes to fungi.

The first commercialised application in 1994, in the United States, by the company Calgene was the "long" preservation transgenic tomato. However, this tomato did not offer satisfactory taste qualities from the consumer's point of view. New research is now employed in improving taste, a high β-carotene content of tomatoes or with respect with melons, an increased sugar content combined with long conservation.

At the same time, research teams and professional groups work on the valorisation of "minor Mediterranean species" of fruits and vegetables, in a conservation of biodiversity and agricultural and food diversification perspective. This process will be backed by systematic identification and assay of micronutrients and micro-constituents, beneficial for the health of consumers of each of these species (figs, pomegranate, arbutus-berry).

Olive oil

The works of epidemiologists and nutritionists (see chapter "Olive oil, olive oil by-products and olive fruit") have established a relationship between olive oil fatty acid content (mostly oleic acid) and non glyceride fractions (anti-oxidant polyphenols), and its "nutritional value".

Thus, the beneficial effect of olive oil with respect to the prevention of cardiovascular disease is related to the combination of oleic acid, recognised as a hypocholesterolemic agent and the anti-oxidant properties reducing LDL (low density lipoproteins) oxidability. Oxidised LDLs play a major role in the atherogenic process.

Research aiming at improving the nutritional properties of olive fruits and olive oils are based on a greater knowledge of phenolic compound composition. This depends on the variety and degree of maturity of the olives at the time of oil expression (extraction). After that inventory phase, the identification of nutritional markers to be taken into account for varietal selection will allow the optimisation of the health value of olives and olive oil, at the same time as their organoleptic qualities.

The comparative advantage of olive oil over other vegetable oils, even issued from genetically modified varieties, is related to its "double anti-oxidant action":

– one "passive", due to the mono-unsaturated fatty acids which are subject to little or no oxidation;

– the other "active" by the presence of polyphenolic anti-oxidants.

Thus, the creation of sunflower varieties with high oleic acid content or rape without erucic acid, the increase in their oil yield and the modification of their poly-unsaturated fatty acid content will not allow these oils to act according to the same nutritional mechanisms as olive oil.

Fresh cheeses and yoghurts

The Mediterranean diet dairy products recommended are limited to fresh cheeses from ewe or goat milk, due to their low saturated fatty acid content in the lipid fraction and their relative richness in unsaturated fatty acids (18: 3 n-3 = linolenic acid (see chapter "Health benefits of the Mediterranean consumption model"). Yoghurts are also recommended due to the nutrients made by the microflora (*Lactobacillus*, lactic bacteria): secretion of proteins, and water soluble vitamins from the B group.

In this field, the hygienic quality of the milk, the comprehension and solving of technological problems *(Listeria monocytogenes, Clostridium butyricum)* and the generalisation of refrigeration have contributed to the improvement of dairy product quality.

Research continues on lactic and propionic flora, as well as surface flora (yeasts, *Penicillium*, *Geotrichum*, *Corynebacterium*, etc.) in microbial genetics, on the stability of the strains used in fermentation and maturing of cheese, and the study of their behaviour during manufacturing (process engineering).

Zootechnical research aims to develop the expression of κ casein, in goats, which conditions the texture of cheese. Furthermore, other research, have as a goal the expression of the human α S1 casein gene in goat milk, to increase its biological value (digestibility). Other studies aim at reducing lactose concentration, suppress β-lactoglobulin expression, which is known to be allergenic in certain sensitive subjects (Leroy, 1997).

Fish

Fish (*see chapter* "Fish and sea foods") overall have a beneficial effect on health and in particular, a protective effect for cardiovascular diseases by the lipids present that have anti-fibrillation properties on cardiac muscle, in relation with the risk of death in the days following a myocardial infarction.

The n-3 series poly-unsaturated fatty acid (EPA, DHA) proportions are also likely to be involved in intra-tumoural necrosis vascular phenomena and to reduce the appearance of metastasis.

Thus, the recommendation to consume fish (*see chapter* "Eating behaviour and culinary practices") is subject to two constraints:

– on the one hand, that of the preservation of fish fatty acids, which are rapidly oxidised after fishing and death of the fish. Therefore, it is essential to rapidly prepare, refrigerate or freeze the fish on the fishing grounds;

– on the other hand, that of the availability of fish stocks which decrease with increasing fishing pressure.

On that level, the development of fish farming will allow:

– an improved management of existing resources, respecting repopulation dynamics;

– a diversification of fished species, subject to the verification of the quality of their nutritional properties;

– a limitation of the attacks on the natural milieu on certain sites and the protection of the environment; combined with selective fishing techniques, thus it could ensure a sustainable production and meet an increasing consumption.

At the European level, fresh water fish farming, with the development of salmonids (rainbow trouts) covers approximately 82% of the requirements. In sea water fish farming, the Mediterranean basin produces 85% of the molluscs (mussels, oysters) consumed in the Mediterranean and close to 15% of the fish (breams, wolffishes and mullets), while the Atlantic basin, North sea and the Baltic, produce 57% of the molluscs and 30% of the fish, especially salmon, a product that used to be considered as a luxury product, and is progressively entering common consumption (Welcomme, 1997).

Thus, while the growth of fishing in Europe is limited for the reasons indicated of overexploitation of stocks of the main species captured, progress in fish farming both in volume and in diversification are significant. In this sense an effort in the search of protein sources adapted to the needs of farmed fish is required. Furthermore, a prevention of the pollution risks, inherent to intensive farming systems, and a protection of the environment and sites should be developed.

With respect to fish preservation, research is carried out on a fast characterisation of freshness, the study of molecular interactions during treatments, especially texturing, and the analysis of new food sources (fish, algae, shellfish).

Thus, the development of efficient sensors, the generation of knowledge on the nutritional interest (constituents, micro-constituents) of new species and their biological properties are a priority in this field.

Poultry and eggs

In agreement with Delpeuch (*see chapter* "Preserve and promote Mediterranean food for health"), eggs and poultry meat contribute, in the context of a judicious combination with practical use quality products, to ensure a diversified diet.

Indeed, if the consumption of red meat may be associated with an increase in the risk of colon cancer, the consumption of poultry, like that of fish, is on the contrary associated with a reduction in this risk (*see chapter* "Health benefits of the Mediterranean consumption model").

Apart from these nutritional aspects, it must be underlined that poultry and eggs are foods widely used and accepted on a cultural level. Fischler (1993) mentions that, out of close to 383 dietary ethnic cultures and traditions studied, poultry was well accepted in 363 of them, which makes it a "universal" food, largely ahead of other animal protein sources (for example 159 for fish, 108 for sheep, according to Abrams, 1987).

New agricultural practices and agro-food innovation

Research perspectives take into account consumer behaviour, price, product diversification that contribute to competition between animal species and producing countries.

Thus, the fat content of poultry carcass and strain prolificacy are the subject of genetic research on a world-wide scale. The slaughtering and carving of poultry must improve their exploitation results that are very low today (close to 0% to 0.5% of turnover at best, both for turkey and chicken).

Wine

Wine and grape by-products have been the subject of numerous studies that aimed at a better understanding of their beneficial and/or undesirable effects on health. While grapes can be assimilated to the global benefit provided by fruits (*see chapter* "Health benefits of the Mediterranean consumption model" and "Beneficial effects of fruits and vegetables on health") or fruit juices, wine consumption must be more closely examined on a benefit/risk ratio level, related to a dose-effect with a threshold established by the alcohol intake.

We will retain, with Claude-Louis Léger (*see chapter* "Wine consumption and cardiovascular disease prevention"), that moderate consumption of wine protects against cardiovascular diseases. It should be added that it is mainly the effects of wine with respect to these risks that have been studied. In a December 1999 review that we carried out concerning 258 scientific publications listed in Medline, 96 were about cardiovascular pathologies.

Cancers, under various forms, and degenerative diseases (of metabolism or central nervous system) have benefited from many fewer publications: 22 and 6, respectively. Thus, apart from research that allows a better setting of alcohol sensitivity thresholds depending on the individuals, related to age or sex, and to predisposition factors, research is oriented towards the anti-oxidant effects and other effects of polyphenols and of their metabolites in humans. Knowledge on their bioavailability, the mechanisms of action of "marker" molecules from the different wine polyphenol families should allow a better evaluation of the role of wine(s), not only in the prevention of cardiovascular diseases, but also with respect to various forms of cancers and degenerative diseases or related to ageing.

TECHNOLOGICAL INNOVATIONS AND TRANSFORMATIONS

In the context of this work, it is a question of identifying in technological innovation matters those that can preserve nutrients and in particular micro-constituents identified as markers of interest for consumer health, by favouring for example their release after transformation and/or ingestion.

Other technologies can increase the health benefit desired. Among "key technologies" such as defined by the GIS (Groupement national d'intérêt scientifique (National scientific interest group)) RIA (recherche sur les industries alimentaires (food industry research)) and developed by its co-ordinator, Pierre Feillet (Feillet, 1998), most can contribute to this objective of ensuring the control of the conception and manufacture of industrially prefabricated foods and drinks.

We will mention first aeraulics, which consists in controlling the particles transported by ambient air flows. The applications aim at the prevention of air contamination sources at a factory or workshop scale (this is the objective of the "ultra-clean factory" program) or equipment and work places. It is then referred to as close protection (for example, using filtered air laminar flow hoods).

Microbial ecology studies the interactions between foods (considered as substrates from this point of view) and beneficial bacterial or fungal flora useful for biotransformation processes or related to saprophytics or pathogenic contaminants (that could induce a technological risk or affect hygienic safety of foods).

The development of methods or means of manufacturing in-process controls should provide instantaneous indications, without massive destruction of the product. These are the fast non-invasive methods and "on-line" sensors. They are widely applied to physical or optical measurements (temperature, relative humidity, water content, pH, particle measurement, colours, etc.).

We are thus heading towards an "assisted" conception of foods, simultaneously taking into account the biochemical, physical, hygienic, nutritional and organoleptic characteristics desired and trying to optimise them, both for the definition of the manufacturing parameters and the in-process and finished product quality control.

With respect to the health value of foods, most frequently "mild" or "minimal" technologies will be chosen, in order to preserve the fresh or "equivalent to fresh" characteristics of finished products, while ensuring their hygienic safety (*see chapter* "Preserve the health capital of food with appropriate technological treatments").

Thus, historically pasteurisation or the use of "ultra-high temperature" for a very limited time for liquid products (milk, juice, etc) met this type of concern.

More recently, the use of high pressure combined with freezing seems promising, under condition of developing equipment that would allow continuous work on an industrial scale.

The application of electrical fields, magnetic fields or pulsed light rays are at an experimental level in the laboratory. They allow the decontamination of bacteria, fungi, spores and viruses on the surface and on products presented under various forms: powders, pasta, and heterogeneous solids. The applications are potentially vast (spices, flours, dehydrated vegetables, egg products, cheese, cold cuts, cooked dishes, etc.). However, industrial developments must validate these new technologies, especially in economic terms.

Other physical processes have been developed successfully and meet this mild technology criterion. Thus, osmotic dehydration or dehydration-impregnation by immersion in a concentrated solution, in order to limit the water content has been successfully applied to fruits, drinks and meat products. Fruit morsels or fish filets preserve good texture and sensory analysis characteristics and a high dry matter content, compatible with a better preservation or transformation.

The knowledge of microbial ecology and enzymatic expression systems also allows the control of microbiological quality of certain foods: it is the case of dairy products and cheeses, using microbial agents that express the lacto-peroxydase system, allowing the inhibition of pathogenic bacteria such as *Listeria* sp.

New agricultural practices and agro-food innovation

Finally, it seems useful to mention that standard technologies, applied to raw materials searched by nutritionists and prescribing physicians, dieticians, but whose consumption was up to now limited as they could not be used simply and practically, may constitute an important innovation for a nutritional approach to diet. It was in this manner that "Ebly" (pre-cooked wheat) was successfully created and meets the objective of developing the daily consumption of cereals.

References

• CFS, GNIS, UIPP. *Les plantes génétiquement modifiées, une clef pour l'avenir*. St-Denis : Imprimerie Rosay, 1997 : 67.

• Champ M. Céréales : aspect nutrition. 8ᵉ Journées Nationales de Diététique (n° spécial) 1997 : 1-6.

• Drewnowski A. Comment évaluer la qualité de l'ensemble du régime alimentaire ? *Cah Nutr Diet* 1999 ; 34(1) : 15-20.

• Feillet P. *Un point sur... aliments et industries alimentaires : les priorités de la recherche publique*. Paris : INRA, 1998 : 288.

• Fischler C. *L'Homnivore : le goût, la cuisine et le corps*. Paris : Odile Jacob, 1993 : 29.

• Labonne G, Quiot JB, Quiot L, Lauriaut F. Enroulement chlorotique de l'abricotier. Identification des vecteurs et lutte. 10ᵉ Rencontres INRA, Agro Montpellier, 1999 : 83-4.

• Leroy P. Amélioration de la production. In : *La Recherche agronomique européenne dans le monde du XXIᵉ siècle : quelle innovation pour l'alimentation, l'agriculture et le cadre de vie ?* Palais de l'Europe. Strasbourg : INRA, Brodard et Taupin, 1997.

• Peyrière J, et al. Amélioration de la compétitivité de la filière salade en Roussillon. 10ᵉ Rencontres INRA-Agro Montpellier, 1999 : 87-8.

• Quiot JB, et al. Lutte contre la sharka : raisonnements et mise en place d'une protection du verger méridional. 10ᵉ Rencontres INRA, Agro Montpellier, 1999 : 85-6.

• Welcomme R. Diversification des productions. In : *La recherche agronomique européenne dans le monde du XXIᵉ siècle : quelle innovation pour l'alimentation, l'agriculture et le cadre de vie ?* Palais de l'Europe. Strasbourg : INRA, Brodard et Taupin, 1997 : 176-81.

Preserving and promoting the Mediterranean diet for health: towards integrated nutrition policies

Francis Delpeuch

Interest in the beneficial effects of the Mediterranean diet for health dates back to the 1950s when Ancel Keys and his wife Margaret undertook epidemiological observations in southern Italy and Greece. This was the first time a link was established between the kind of food usually eaten in these regions, which is notably low in fats, and one of the highest life expectancy rates in the world together with some of the lowest rates of chronic disease, particularly coronary disease. When the results of the famed "seven countries study" confirmed this link, a previously unknown concept, the "Mediterranean Diet", was born.

If the term has now taken its place, with positive connotations, in both everyday language and in the scientific literature, its exact definition is often unclear. It generally refers to the food traditionally eaten in the countries that border the Mediterranean or in certain regions of those countries. Over and above the many national and regional variations (*see chapter* "Eating Behavior and Culinary Practices"), the main characteristic all these diets had in common was that their main component was plant foods, *i.e.* cereals, often only partially refined, legumes, a considerable variety of fruits and vegetables, a wide range of aromatic herbs, olive oil as the main source of fat, and wine, drunk in moderate quantities with meals. However, this by no means implies that the diets were vegetarian: cheese, mainly made from goat's and sheep's milk, and fish and meat were consumed to a varying extent, often as a side dish, in almost all the regions concerned, and traditional Mediterranean food has always been appreciated both for its taste and its hedonistic qualities. But it should also be emphasized that the diets were relatively frugal with no excess calories, and were also an integral part of a lifestyle that included regular physical exercise and that consequently resulted in low rates of obesity in the populations concerned.

From the nutritional point of view, the main observation made at that time was the low fat content of the diet, particularly saturated fatty acids. Interest in Mediterranean food resurfaced when results of both epidemiological and experimental studies demonstrated the importance of oxidative stress in chronic and degenerative diseases, as well as the previously unrecognized anti-oxidizing capacity of certain vitamins, minerals and biologically active substances, for example polyphenols and flavonoids *(see Technical information)*. These substances, which are currently the subject of intense research, occur in many of the plant foods that characterize the Mediterranean diet.

Thus today, the Mediterranean diet would appear to have a double nutritional advantage in the prevention of chronic disease:

– It contains fewer harmful components, for example fewer excess saturated fatty acids;

– It contains more protective components: anti-oxidants, folates and fibers among others.

This new scientific knowledge enables us to formulate a number of recommendations for a diet for improved health and general well-being *(see Parts I and II of this book)*.

TRADITIONAL MEDITERRANEAN DIET:
A GOOD MODEL FOR HEALTHY EATING

In the 1990s, what was described as the "Traditional Mediterranean Diet" – among the many variations found in Mediterranean food – was considered to be the most beneficial for health (see box'Characteristics of the traditional Mediterranean diet). This was the diet that could still be found in the south of Italy, in Crete and in most regions of Greece at the beginning of the 1960s, regions that also had the highest life expectancy rates and the lowest rates of chronic disease (Milio & Helsing, 1998; Trichopoulou & Lagiou, 1997; Willet *et al.*, 1995).

This was also the beginning of the concept of the Mediterranean diet pyramid as a cultural model for a healthy eating (Willet *et al.*, 1995) *(figure 1)*. This type of model offers an innovative way of informing and educating the general public about food and nutrition (Milio, Helsing, 1998) as an alternative to the more traditional approach that simply provided theoretical nutritional guidelines, an approach whose usefulness has been shown to be limited. Rather than trying to enforce precise instructions that in practice are very difficult to respect, the diet pyramid allows for a very wide choice in the type and quantity of food as well as how often it can be consumed. The principle underlying the elaboration of this model was the identification of diets and lifestyles that, in a given period and a given context, have been linked to populations who enjoy exceptionally good health. The research that goes into the creation of models of this type includes health, nutrition (both epidemiological and biological) as well as diet, culture, history and culinary traditions.

The **Mediterranean Diet Pyramid** presents a diet than can be followed by the majority of adults. For use in nutrition education, certain adjustments probably need to be made, particularly concerning pregnancy and breast-feeding, as well as for young children, who have specific growth requirements, and perhaps also for other segments of the population.

The pyramid in its exact form is not necessarily to be recommended throughout the world. Other regions, for example Asia, have traditional cultural lifestyles that correspond to international dietary recommendations. However it has been proposed as a general framework that could encourage healthful changes in eating habits in North America as well as in northern and in eastern Europe, and in the United States it is the basis of current dietary recommendations. In Europe, the same dietary structure as that proposed by the pyramid could be

> **Characteristics of the traditional Mediterranean diet**
>
> 1) An abundance of plant foods including fresh fruits and vegetables, potatoes, bread and other grains, beans, legumes and dried fruits;
> 2) A wide variety of minimally processed foods, and, wherever possible, locally grown food that is in season (optimization of micro-nutriments and anti-oxidants);
> 3) Olive oil as the main source of fat rather than other types of oil and fat (including butter and margarine);
> 4) A maximum of 7-8% of energy provided by saturated fats, with total fat ranging between 25 and 35% of energy;
> 5) Daily consumption of small quantities of cheese and yoghurt (products with low or no fat content may be preferred);
> 6) Weekly consumption of small to medium quantities of fish and poultry (recent research suggests that the consumption of fish could be encouraged) and up to 4 eggs (including those in prepared foods);
> 7) Daily consumption of fresh fruit, as the typical dessert; consumption of sweet foods with significant amounts of sugar and saturated fats not more than a few times a week;
> 8) Red meat only eaten a few times per month (recent research suggests that consumption should be limited to 340-450g per month, where the flavor is acceptable, lean versions may be preferred);
> 9) Regular physical activity to promote a healthy weight, fitness and wellbeing;
> 10) Moderate consumption of wine, generally at meals, 1-2 glasses per day for men and 1 glass per day for women. The consumption of wine should be considered optional and be avoided whenever consumption would put the individual and others at risk, for example during pregnancy or in situations when vigilance is required.
>
> *(Adapted from Milio & Helsing, 1998)*

obtained using dishes typical of other regions than those located around the Mediterranean. In the Mediterranean region it could be used to maintain traditional Mediterranean diets and their advantages while adapting them to changes in lifestyles.

Beyond these considerations, can and should recommendations be made based on any one isolated factor?

Concerning nutriments and particularly antioxidants, results of the most recent studies (presented in the chapters entitled "Health benefits of the Mediterranean consumption model" and "Olive oil, olive oil by-products and olive fruit: current data and developments concerning the food and health relationship") show that there is neither one miracle molecule nor a single solution for optimal nutrition. It would be very risky to develop new varieties (of olive trees or vines, for example) based on such assumptions when everything tends to indicate that the answer is to be found in the diversity of plant varieties as well as in the effect of the soil, in other words, in the wealth of resources in nature. On the other hand it would seem perfectly justified to continue to study:

– variations in content in different products (of a particular anti-oxidant, for example) and more especially the associations that exist;

– food processing, to conserve quality and to manufacture products that are practical to use.

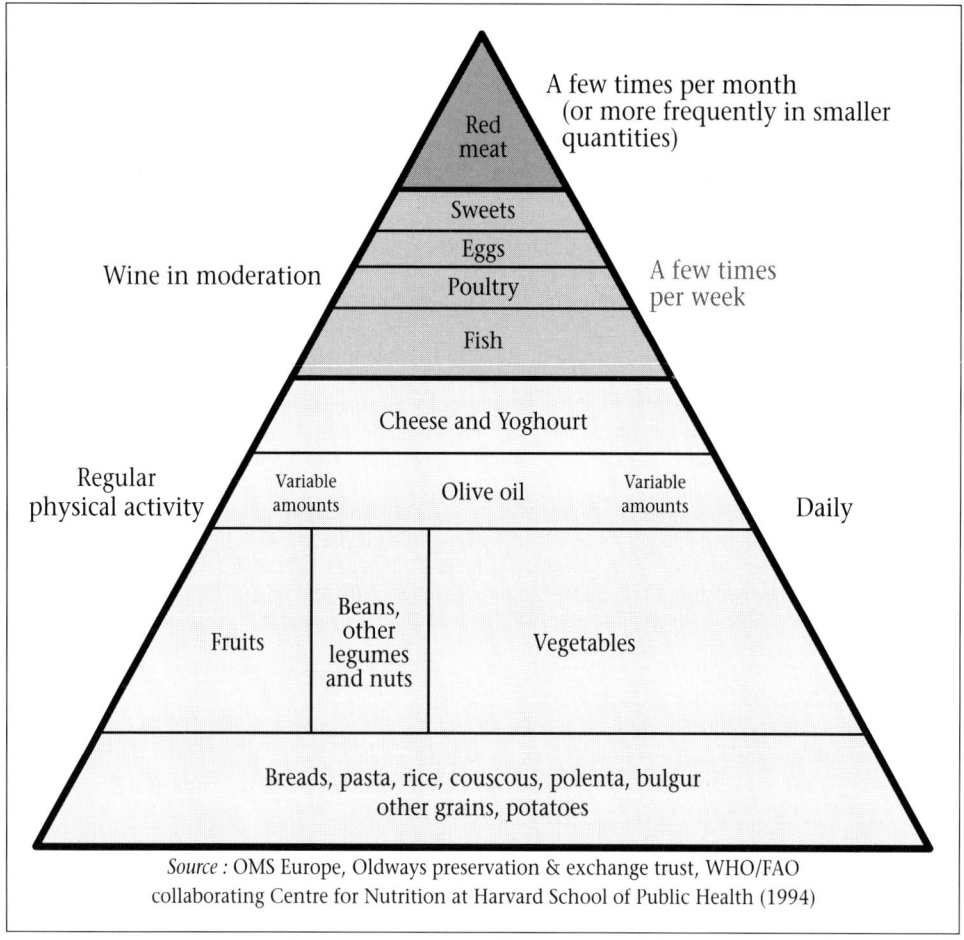

Figure 1. The Mediterranean Diet Pyramid: a traditional model for a healthy diet and lifestyle.

Concerning food, research findings are the same: there can be no "food effect" isolated from nutrition as a whole. The results of the studies given in the first two parts of this book are in agreement with the lessons that can be drawn from observations of various aspects of Mediterranean diet that are described in *Part III*: "Eating behavior and culinary practices". What is striking is the enormous variety of cooking techniques, the different practices, the range of know-how and the different types of food used. Thus there is practically no specific food item that stands out, what is specific is the way the items are combined, the seasonal variations and the way the food is eaten.

Wine provides one of the best examples of the need to consider nutrition as a "whole" when considering the benefits of the Mediterranean diet for health. Drunk in moderate quantities with meals, wine is clearly part of the Mediterranean diet; nevertheless, consumption must be considered optional as it can have a number of undesirable effects (*see box* "Characteristics of the Mediterranean Diet"). Thus we cannot make isolated recommendations that could legitimize excess consumption or even lead those who do not drink wine to think that they should.

Assuming we accept the advantages of considering the Mediterranean diet as a whole, there are a number of questions concerning the countries in the Mediterranean region that require urgent answers: what does the term "Mediterranean diet" really mean today? How can it be preserved or how can a trend that is frequently considered to be unfavorable be reversed? Or to go even further, perhaps what we are talking about is a whole new way of looking at nutrition, right along the food chain, and including its long-term consequences for health.

WHEN FACED WITH CHANGE, SHOULD WE LOOK TO THE PAST OR PROMOTE NEW IDEAS?

There are many indications that for the past few years lifestyles and diets have been becoming more uniform in Europe. In Italy and Crete the consumption of meat, dairy products and animal fats has increased considerably since the 1960s while the consumption of bread, fruit and even olive oil decreased over the same period (Nestle, 1995). In many countries in the region some data suggest that these changes in eating habits are being accompanied by a general decrease in physical activity and by an increase in the rate of obesity, in high rates of cholesterol and in high blood pressure, resulting in an increase in the incidence of coronary diseases, diabetes and certain cancers linked to nutrition. The significance of these changes is the subject of controversy: some think that the Mediterranean diet is in danger and that its advantages for health are being questioned even in Mediterranean countries themselves (Nestle, 1995); others believe that its basic characteristics have been maintained despite recent changes and that the comparative advantages this diet offers in terms of vital statistics are still just as obvious (for example in southern Italy: Ferro-Luzzi & Branca, 1995).

Generally speaking, with respect to the benefits for health mentioned above, Mediterranean countries have experienced both negative changes - an increase in the consumption of products of animal origin, a decrease in the consumption of cereals, particularly partially refined cereals, and of legumes, and positive changes - an increase in the consumption of fruits.

Thus, depending on the context, it may be necessary to reverse a trend or simply to conserve favorable factors. But aside from these changes, it is also important to remember that at the beginning of the 1960s, the combination of factors that made up the traditional Mediterranean model that is most beneficial for health (presented in *figure 1*) was only found in a very limited part of the Mediterranean region. If, in the search for improved health and well-being, the aim is to approach the model as closely as possible, this by no means implies returning to eating habits and life-styles that may be outdated, but to look ahead in adopting a healthier diet and way of life. Of course, this would – in theory at least – be much easier to achieve in Mediterranean countries where existing diets are generally much closer to the traditional Mediterranean model than are diets in northern European countries.

Today, everyone agrees that many different cultural, social, economic and institutional factors influence diet in the Mediterranean region as they do elsewhere, and that if diet does have a major influence on health, other factors also have to be taken into consideration. The changes that have been observed in Spain over the last two decades, referred to the "Spanish paradox" after the famous "French paradox", are a perfect illustration of the complexity of the links between diet and health as well as the significance of non-dietary factors (Serra-Majem et al., 1995). As a matter of fact, in Spain the mortality rate due to heart disease has decreased consistently since 1976 although the consumption of meat, dairy products, fruit and fish has increased and the consumption of olive oil, sugar and foods rich in complex carbohydrates has decreased. Thus despite a significant increase in the consumption of fats and particularly of saturated fats, there has been no accompanying increase in deaths due to coronary heart disease. This paradox can perhaps be explained by the increase in the consumption of fruits and of fish and also to wider access to health care as well as improved monitoring for hypertension and a decrease in smoking.

> A recent study showed that during the period from 1992 to 1996, the mean per capita consumption of fruit and vegetables in Spain was 600g per day; this figure is much higher than in the majority of other European countries and approximately double that observed in France and the USA during the same period. (Agudo et al., 1999).

The wide variety of contexts and sectors involved naturally leads us to the conclusion that the survival of the Mediterranean diet in the region where it was born and its extension to other regions will depend on the creation and implementation of global nutrition policies.

GLOBAL, INTEGRATED FOOD AND NUTRITION POLICIES

A nutrition policy can be defined as a combination of concerted actions based on scientific principles that aims firstly to ensure that all segments of the population have access to supplies of safe, good quality, correctly labeled food at affordable prices, and secondly to promote and facilitate the consumption of food that is good for health (Milio & Helsing, 1998). They relate to all sector policies concerned with food – to a greater or lesser extent – that need to pay more attention to the health and nutritional well-being of the population when defining their objectives.

These policies are global to the extent that they deal with both supply (production, processing, distribution) and demand (consumer choice). To promote further development of the Mediterranean diet with the objective of preventing disease and promoting health, nutrition policies must provide answers to three main questions (O'Brien, 1995):

– How can we encourage a wide range in the choice of food?

– How can we facilitate, if required, corresponding changes in the agricultural sector?

– How can we strengthen the contribution made by processed products?

Integration emphasizes the importance of cooperation and coordination between the different sectors involved at the national and local level, the complementarity of agricultural policies and public health policies, and the need for the agri-food industry to support and respect these policies.

The concept of food and nutrition policies is not new, but from the 1950s until the 1980-1990s, these policies were primarily quantitative (the aim was to produce sufficient quantities of food) and questions were mainly concerned with producers and self-sufficiency. A study carried out in 21 countries in the 1980s showed that not one food policy had nutritional objectives (WHO, 1990). In Europe, only Norway and Finland had explicit nutrition policies and these were based on links between diet and chronic and degenerative diseases. Nevertheless, as early as 1951, the first FAO/WHO expert committee on nutrition declared that there was good reason to believe that excessive consumption particularly of sugar and fats could lead to serious forms of malnutrition (Helsing, 1997). This idea, which was innovative at the time, was far from the priorities and nutritional criteria that dominated the immediate post-war period and permanently shaped agriculture and the food industry in Europe and the USA and that are now outdated (Delpeuch & Maire, 1996). Today these priorities and criteria are still just as far from the principles that underlie the benefits for health of the Mediterranean diet. They were partly responsible for the drift towards overproduction in the agricultural and food industry that has been strongly criticized during the last few years, and obviously need reviewing in the light of relevant scientific criteria and given today's social needs. In 1990 the WHO study group on diet, nutrition and the prevention of chronic disease drew attention to the relevance of this particular question for Europe:

"Agricultural and economic policies, which are naturally linked to those of the European Economic Community, are not necessarily compatible with existing knowledge on diet and health" (WHO, 1990).

The idea expressed by the expert committee in 1951 found little echo and it took 40 years for it to gradually find acceptance. Things began to change in Europe when the first intergovernment conference on world nutrition (International Conference on Nutrition – ICN – Rome, 1992) adopted a holistic approach to questions concerning diet and nutrition. This stimulated the majority of countries to draw up national plans of action that were the true precursors of today's nutrition policies.

As early as 1994, of the 33 countries that comprise Europe (as defined by the WHO), 28 had prepared a plan of action for nutrition. The three most frequent strategies were:

– improvement in the food quality and safety;

– promotion of appropriate diets and healthy lifestyles;

– assessment, analysis and monitoring of nutrition situations.

Eighteen countries also adopted as one of their strategies the incorporation of nutritional objectives into development policies and programs.

In this context, Mediterranean countries now find themselves in a paradoxical situation with regard to change. Traditionally in these countries there has been little political interest or concern about problems of public health linked to diet. This paradox may be explained by the favorable circumstances in which the countries found themselves in terms of vital statistics and risk factors in comparison with northern countries.

A number of characteristics shared by northern countries have also been brought to light and should be taken into consideration in the implementation of nutrition policies:

– recommendations about diet that are often unrealistic or ill-adapted to the real context of the population;

– over-medicalization of actions, little emphasis on the food supply and consequently on the food chain;

– overconfidence in the virtues of the Mediterranean diet, which could lead, for example, to over-consumption of olive oil, wine or dried fruits, for example;

– lack of coordination between the health and agricultural sectors;

– various legislative problems (Serra-Majem *et al.*, 1997).

IMPLEMENTATION OF NUTRITION POLICIES

Two principles govern the formulation of nutrition policies:

– one solution is never enough;

– the combination of strategies and measures required will vary with the context.

A general framework (major options, main stages, institutional aspects) for the development of nutrition policies in Europe has been described elsewhere (Milio & Helsing, 1998). However we think it would be useful to emphasize several key points with respect to the aim of conserving and promoting the Mediterranean diet.

Inter-sectoral considerations are at the forefront, as underlined by the plan of action proposed by the ICN:

"Improved nutrition requires the coordinated efforts of relevant government ministries, agencies and offices with mandates for agriculture, fisheries and livestock, food, health water and public works, supplies, planning, finance, industry, education, information, social welfare and trade. It also requires the cooperation of universities and research institutions; food producers, processors and marketers; the health care community; educators at all levels; the media and NGOs involved in all of these sectors" (ICN, 1992).

It is necessary to take into account the range of different interests at stake, as well as a certain consensus between the different sectors involved, even though the main objective remains health and well-being. One of the pre-conditions for success is the existence of a central facility that will allow the exchange of ideas and manage the multi-factorial nature of the problem, where different institutions would normally be in charge. An advisory body would seem to provide the best solution to:

– evaluate, analyze and monitor the situation;

– define general guidelines and propose priority actions;

– monitor their implementation in liaison with the different public and private sectors concerned;

– prepare the modifications required as a result of advances in knowledge or the appearance of new technologies.

The scope of nutrition policies is vast because it includes everything that influences food supply and demand. Thus many different measures are possible.

Food demand: consumer choice

Informing and educating the public about the links between diet and health is a long-term task that require a permanent investment in effort and must be accompanied by nutrition training programs aimed at people in all branches of the medical profession and education, as well as those in charge of institutional kitchens and food production. Dietary recommendations and the nutritional information on food labels also helps the public to choose a wider range of healthy, good quality food from an increasingly complex supply.

Food supply: agricultural production, processing and distribution of products, institutional food in the public and private sector

Despite growing awareness among consumers of the link between diet and health, the ability and/or the will to change may be limited or may take a long time. Regulations applying to the supply of food (legislation, standards for quality and hygiene, inspections) have frequently proved useful if not indispensable, and there is no reason to believe that the promotion of the Mediterranean diet will be any different. The modification of the characteristics of certain food products is a potential way to increase their nutritional value and to reduce their defects. For example in the treatment of deficiencies in micronutrients such as iron, iodine or vitamin A, fortification programs have already proved useful. However, the prevention of chronic disease is much more complex. Finally, economic measures concerning the production and consumption of food should not be excluded.

The perception and the point of view of the general public must be taken into consideration in the choice of components of nutrition policies. However, a recent study showed that in Europe, quality, price and flavor are the main factors influencing consumers' choice of food (Robertson, 1998); and food safety is perceived to be the biggest problem for health despite the fact that, in the European context, all scientific data indicate that an unbalanced diet has much more serious long-term consequences for health. Should we consequently cry victory and limit our actions to ensuring food safety and low prices, or to the contrary, place emphasis on actions that foster a more informed and responsible choice by consumers?

All the above-mentioned actions can, either directly or indirectly, via changes in consumer choices, lead to changes in the agricultural sector and in the food industry as a whole (Johnson, 1994). This is why close collaboration between the two sectors is so important, not only for reasons of efficiency, but also so that changes will not be perceived as a threat, but to the contrary, as an opportunity for innovation and increased competitive effectiveness.

Finally, one important pre-condition for success is the existence of nutrition surveillance activities that would provide regular, pertinent and high quality information on diet and on the nutritional status of the population concerned, as well as on the principal factors responsible for that status (Maire et al, 1999).

In conclusion, it is true to say that we are all aware of policies, programs and measures that could contribute, globally or more specifically, to the development of nutrition policies. What remains to be done is to determine, in each particular case, the best possible combination of policies and programs for a whole country or for a specific region.

On this last point, geopolitical changes in Europe have presented us with a new configuration in the form of two new developments: firstly the transfer of responsibility from the State to the European Parliament and to the European Commission - agricultural policy being one of the key examples, and secondly, decentralization with the transfer of responsibilities that previously belonged to central governments to the regions. After the ICN, the Spanish central government mandated the regions and provided the resources to handle questions concerning health and nutrition. As part of its health plan, Catalonia has drawn up the first nutrition policy in Spain (see box), and this policy is considered to be a model for the other Spanish regions (Serra-Majem et al., 1997).

Between common policies and specific regional policies, the European institutional landscape is becoming progressively more complex and more diversified. Further studies are indispensable, but this diversity already offers a wide range of opportunities to develop – in harmony with general changes in health policies concerning disease prevention and the promotion of health – innovative nutrition policies that promote the Mediterranean diet and the improvements in health and well-being that everybody now concedes it can produce.

Spanish Catalonia: an example of a regional nutrition policy

Main steps in establishing priorities:
– careful analysis of main public health problems in terms of mortality, morbidity, disability, economic and social costs; estimation of the incidence and of the potential consequences of risk factors for chronic disease;
– examination of the benefits and of the political, institutional and financial feasibility of different actions likely to reduce health problems and risk factors;
– identification of priorities based on the preceding points. Among the 13 health problems identified, the first 6 are directly related to eating habits. Among the 18 courses of action selected, those connected with food rank third.

Some characteristics of the Catalonian nutrition policy:
– objectives were defined for food and nutrition;
– dietary recommendations are diffused to health centers;
– contractualisation is underway, particularly concerning preventive actions targeting highly ranked health problems, and including continuing education of staff involved in primary health care;
– although the health sector is predominant (in this case nutrition policy is an integral part of the health plan), the importance of other sectors (*e.g.* agriculture, economy, industry and commerce, the environment, etc.) is recognized and their participation appears to be genuine;
– the existence of nutrition surveillance activities including an overall evaluation of the nutritional status of the Catalonian population, follow-up of dietary objectives and implementation of actions.

Adapted from Serra-Majem et al., 1997

References

- Rapport final de la Conférence Internationale sur la nutrition. FAO, OMS, Rome, 1992 : 63 p.

- Delpeuch F, Maire B. Situation nutritionnelle dans le monde : changements et enjeux. *Cahiers Agricultures* 1996 ; 5 : 415-22.

- EPIC Group of Spain : Agudo, *et al*. Dietary intake of vegetables and fruits among adults in five regions of Spain. *Eur J Clin Nutr* 1999 ; 53(3) : 174-80.

- Ferro-Luzzi A, Branca F. Mediterranean diet, Italian-style : prototype of a healthy diet. *Am J Clin Nutr* 1995 ; 61(6 Suppl.) : 1338S-1345S.

- Helsing E. The history of nutrition policy. *Nutr Rev* 1997 ; 55(11 Pt 2) : S1-S3.

- Johnson SR. How nutrition policy affects food and agricultural policy. *J Nutr* 1994 ; 124 (9 Suppl) : 1871S-1877S.

- Keys A. Coronary heart disease in seven countries. *Circulation* 1970 ; 41 (Suppl. 1) : 1-211.

- Maire B, Beghin I, Delpeuch F, Kolsteren P, Remaut de Winter AM. La surveillance nutritionnelle : une approche opérationnelle et durable. Studies in Health Services Organisation & Policy. Antwerp : ITG Press 1999 ; 13.

- Milio N, Helsing E. European food and nutrition policies in action. WHO regional publications, European Series, 1998 ; n° 73. World Health Organization Regional Office for Europe. Copenhagen, 176 p.

- Nestle M. Mediterranean diets : historical and research overview. *Am J Clin Nutr* 1995 ; 61 (6 Suppl.) : 1313S-1320S.

- O'Brien P. Dietary shifts and implications for US agriculture. *Am J Clin Nutr* 1995 ; 61 (6 Suppl.) : 1390S-1396S.

- OMS. Régime alimentaire, nutrition et prévention des maladies chroniques : rapport d'un Groupe d'étude de l'OMS. Série de Rapports Techniques, 1990 ; n° 797, OMS, Genève, 229 p.

- Robertson A. Health, food, and nutrition policy. *Public Health Rev* 1998 ; 26(1) : 107-8.

- Serra-Majem L, Ferro-Luzzi A, Bellizzi M, Salleras L. Nutrition policies in Mediterranean Europe. *Nutr Rev* 1997 ; 55 (11 Pt 2) : S42-S57.

- Serra-Majem L, Ribas L, Tresserras R, Ngo J, Salleras L. How could changes in diet explain changes in coronary heart disease mortality in Spain ? The Spanish paradox. *Am J Clin Nutr* 1995 ; 61 (6 Suppl.) : 1351S-1359S.

- Trichopoulou A, Lagiou P. Healthy traditional Mediterranean diet : an expression of culture, history, and lifestyle. *Nutr Rev* 1997 ; 55 (11 Pt 1) : 383-9.

- Willett WC, Sacks F, Trichopoulou A, Drescher G, Ferro-Luzzi A, Helsing E, Trichopoulos D. « Mediterranean diet pyramid : a cultural model for healthy eating. » *Am J Clin Nutr* 1995 ; 61 (6 Suppl.) : 1402S-1406S.

Glossary

α-linolenic acid: polyunsaturated fatty acid of the n-3 series, not synthezised by the body (so called essential) and mainly present in plants.

α-tocopherol: vitamin E.

Adenomas: benign tumours.

Agonist: capable of stimulating an endo- or exocrine secretion.

Amylated hydrocarbons: polysaccharides principally composed of starch.

Antagonist: capable of inhibiting an endo- or exocrine secretion.

Anti-hypercholesterolemic (effect...): average (so called normal) cholesterolemia (or plasma cholesterol levels) in adults is of the order of 2.15 g/l. Real hypercholesterolemia starts from 2.5 g/l. An anti-hypercholesterolemic effect defines the action of a substance that opposes hypercholesterolemia, and thus tends to keep cholesterolemia within a so-called normal value range.

Anti-fibrillation effect: myocardial fibrillation is one of the aspects of heart disease.

Atheroma: anatomical-pathological signature of arteriosclerosis. The atheromatous plaque that makes arterial walls rigid, is made up of foam cells (macrophages that phagocytised oxidised LDL).

β-glycuronidase: enzyme capable of deconjugated glycuronated compounds.

BMI: body mass index, as its names indicates, gives the mass of the body taking into account both the weight and height. It is calculated by dividing the weight in kg by the square of the height in meters: thus, a subject weighing 70 kg and measuring 1.80 m will not have the same BMI than a subject weighing 70 kg and measuring 1.65 m (21.6 BMI, normal, and 25,5 BMI, overweight).

Butyrate: short chain fatty acid synthezised by the colon bacterial flora from a polysaccharide substrate.

Carcinogenic: factor of varying nature likely to induce a cancer process.

Carbonyl-amine: bond between a carbon atom and an amine group.

Carotenoids: large family of hydrocarbon compounds, carotenes, including some with oxygen, xantophylls. In our diet the most common carotenes are lycopenes, α- and β-carotene,

Glossary

and the most common xanthophylls are β-cryptoxanthine, luteine and zeaxanthine. α- and β-carotene and β-cryptoxanthine are provitamins A.

Cholesteryl-ester transferase: enzyme involved in HDL cholesterol metabolism.

Cohort: population sample presenting one or several common characteristics that are the subject of a prospective or retrospective epidemiological study, for example women of the MGEN, employees of the French Gas Company.

Confidence interval: statistical calculations take into account possible errors in the measurement of exposure to risk factor and also normal individual variations. For this reason, an estimated relative risk is always accompanied by a range of values that gives the probability limits, this is the confidence interval.

Cruciferae: plant family, including cabbages and chicories, characterised by a flower in the shape of a cross.

Daidzein: an isoflavone from the flavonoid family.

DHA: polyunsaturated fatty acid of the n-3 series, docosohexaenoic acid.

Dose-response effect: there is linear relation between the exposure (dose) and the effect observed (response), for example, the greater the consumption of fruits and vegetables, the lower the risk of developing a cancer of the upper respiratory and digestive tracts.

EPA: polyunsaturated fatty acid of the n-3 series, eicosapentaenoic acid.

Ex vivo **(measurement...):** the measurement of an *ex vivo* biological parameter consists in taking a representative sample (of plasma for example) *in vivo* and then carry out the measurements of this parameter *in vitro*. There may be intermediate separation and purification steps between these two stages.

Ferritin: iron transport protein.

Fibrinogen: protein involved in the formation of blood clots.

Flavonoids: family of natural polyphenolic compounds, including flavonols, flavanols and anthocyanines.

Folic acid: or folates or vitamin B9.

Fatty acids: fat or lipid constituents, made up of polycarbon chains. Their bonds may be saturated or unsaturated. In the latter case the polycarbon chain has double bonds.

Fenton's reaction: reaction in which a transition metal (most often iron) takes part in a chemical reaction leading to the production of hydroxyl radical.

Free radicals: chemical species that have an odd number of electrons with a form particularly favourable to oxidation.

Genistein: an isoflavonol from the flavonoid family.

Haeme iron: iron bound to special proteins such as haemoglobin and myoglobin.

HDL: abbreviation of high density lipoproteins. They are considered to be the good cholesterol transporters.

Glossary

HDL-cholesterol: or "good cholesterol" associated with high density lipoproteins that transport it outside cells.

Heterocyclic aromatic amines: chemical substances in which the cycle is composed of carbon atoms combined with other atoms (O, N, etc.).

Homocysteine: intermediate product on the methionine metabolic path, whose accumulation takes place when there is folate deficiency.

Humoral lipid parameters: components measured in blood that are involved in lipid metabolism: total cholesterol, LDL- and HDL-cholesterol, triglycerides, etc.

Hydroxyl radical: highly oxidant OH- radical

Hydroxytyrosol: phenolic compound present in olive oil.

In vitro: experiment carried out in a test tube, or in a cell culture model, having a limited number of parameters controlled by the investigator.

In vivo: experiment carried out in animals using physiological metabolic paths; *ex vivo*: a dietary experiment or manipulation carried out in humans, and one of the components of the body that is being specifically studied (for example, LDL particles) is taken and introduced in an *in vitro* model.

Ischemic accident: "attack" in popular language or brain softening. From an anatomical-pathological point of view, it corresponds to a zone that has been deprived of vascularisation for a certain amount of time.

Kaempferol: flavonol from the flavonoid family.

LDL-cholesterol: or "bad cholesterol" associated with low density lipoproteins that transport it inside cells.

LDL: abbreviation of low density lipoproteins. They are considered to be the bad cholesterol transporters.

Lignan: plant phyto-oestrogen precursor.

Lipase: enzyme that hydrolyses lipids.

Lipids: fats.

Lipo-oxygenase: enzyme of the metabolic path of arachidonic acid that forms leukotrienes.

Membrane lipids: lipids contained in cellular membranes.

Mesothelioma: special form of lung cancer, situated at the pleura.

Metastases: formation of secondary tumours by dissemination of malignant cells from a primary tumour.

Methionine: sulphated amino acid.

Molybdenum: mineral trace element.

Necrosis: cellular death.

Glossary

NO: nitric acid, smooth muscle relaxant factor.

n-3 fatty acids: polyunsaturated fatty acids that have their first double bond on the 3rd carbon atom on the polycarbon chain.

n-6 fatty acids: polyunsaturated fatty acids that have their first double bond on the 6th carbon atom on the polycarbon chain.

Oestrogen: major sexual hormone present in women. *Oestradiol* and *oestrone*, oestrogen metabolites.

Oestrogen receptor: cellular structure capable of specifically binding oestrogens. There are several forms, including the α receptor (present in mammary tissue and ovaries), and β receptor (also present in mammary tissue but also in other body tissues, bones, brain, vascular wall).

Oleuropein: phenolic compound present in olive oil.

Oxidative stress: oxidative type cellular attack.

Phase I enzymes: they are for the most part the cytochromes, they participate in numerous metabolic reactions in the body, but they are also capable of activating pro-carcinogens into carcinogens.

Phase II enzymes: they participate in numerous detoxification reactions and therefore, are capable of eliminating carcinogens.

Phenolic compounds: chemical compounds comprising one or several phenolic structures that confer on them an anti-oxidant capacity.

PGH synthetase: enzyme of the arachidonic acid metabolic path that synthesises prostaglandins.

Phyto-oestrogens: compounds that have a structure similar to that of human oestrogens but are derived from plant products, mainly isoflavonoids and lignans.

Phospholipase: enzyme that hydrolyses phospholipids.

Platelet aggregation: physico-chemical phenomenon that allows the formation of blood clots.

Pro-oxidant: compound or mechanism capable of inducing oxidative stress.

Quercetin: flavonol from the flavonoid family.

Saturated fats: fatty acids without double bonds.

Triglycerides: glycerol and fatty acid esters.

Tyrosine kinase: enzyme involved in cellular proliferation.

Xenobiotics: compounds not found in living matter, generally chemical contaminants introduced by food.

Index

A

Agro-food innovations 139.
Amino acids 31, 97, 100, 131, 133, 134, 136, 140, 163.
Analytical epidemiology 3.
Anti-nutritional factors 94, 100, 131, 134.
Anti-oxidant properties 27, 59, 60, 80, 89, 94, 95, 97, 142.
Antioxidants 8-11, 13, 20, 22, 26-29, 35, 37, 53, 56, 59-65, 72, 78, 82, 83, 86-89, 94-96, 100, 124, 131, 136, 141, 142, 145, 150, 151, 164.
Atherogenic process 56, 62, 79, 142.
Atheroma 13, 56, 79, 82, 87, 89, 161.
Atherosclerosis 42, 56, 61, 64, 78, 82, 87-89.

B

Beta-carotene 6, 11-13, 20-24, 28, 29, 94, 142, 161, 162.
Bioavailability
of polyphenols 83.
β-sitosterol 58.
Butter 9, 33, 34, 36, 42, 119, 140, 151.

C

Calori intake 9, 35.
Cancer 5-10, 14-34, 36, 38, 39, 57, 64, 69, 70, 93, 109, 141, 144, 145, 153, 161-163.
Complex carbohydrates 94, 154.
Cardiovascular diseases 7, 9-13, 29, 30, 32, 33, 35-39, 54, 69, 70, 77, 78, 82, 87, 88, 93, 94, 96, 110, 113, 126, 141-143, 145.
Cardiovascular risk 11, 14, 37, 54-56, 70, 77-81, 110.
Carotenoids 8, 11, 15, 19-24, 27, 94, 95, 134, 136, 161.
Case-control studies
– intervention 4-6, 12, 13, 17, 18, 20, 22, 28, 29.
– prospective 4, 10, 13, 16-18, 22-25, 27, 28, 30, 31, 36.
Cataract 9, 29, 65.
Cellulose 97-99.
Cereals
– refined 17, 153.
– whole 17, 97, 99, 140.
Cheese 9, 33, 34, 118-120, 123, 133, 139, 143, 146, 149, 151.
Cholesterol 7, 10, 13, 30, 32, 33, 35-39, 54-56, 58, 78, 88, 97, 100, 110, 140, 153, 161-163.
Cholesterolemia 30, 35, 37, 54, 55, 78, 110, 161.
Cognitive ageing 9, 29.
Coumestanes 97.

Index

Culinary practices 111, 113-115, 120, 140, 141, 143, 149, 152.
Cultivars 59.
Cysteine 100, 134, 136.

D

Daidzein 27, 97, 104, 162.
Descriptive epidemiology 3.
Dietary behaviours 37, 116.
Diet quality index (DQI) 140.
Digestive tract 14, 38, 94, 98, 141, 162.

E

Endothelium 79.
Enzyme inhibitors 99, 100, 133.

F

Fatty acids
– polyunsaturated 35, 56, 69, 70, 71, 74, 75, 100, 134, 143, 161, 162, 164.
– saturated 34, 54, 55, 56, 71, 143, 150.
Fibres 101.
– insoluble 98, 100, 109.
– main sources 17, 109.
– physiological 109.
– total dietary 98, 109.
– soluble 11, 98, 100, 109, 110.
Fish 9, 30, 32, 33, 69-76, 114, 120, 122, 123, 139, 140, 143, 144, 146, 149, 151, 154.
Flavanols 22, 82-86, 104, 105, 162.
Flavanones 104, 105.
Flavones 59, 61, 64, 104, 105.
Flavonoid family 104, 162-164.
Foam cells 79, 161.
Folic acid 6, 13, 94, 95, 162.
Food diversity score (FDS) 140
Food health safety 136.
Food variety score (FVS) 140
Free radicals 30, 32, 79, 81, 162.
Free radical scavengers 59, 61, 82, 95.
Fruits 7-11, 13-17, 19, 20, 22, 28, 29, 35, 36, 53, 58, 65, 82, 93-96, 100, 101, 104, 105, 109, 110, 113-115, 119, 120, 123, 139-142, 145, 146, 149, 151, 153, 154, 156, 162.

G

Gall bladder 57.
Gamma-glutamyl-transferase (GGT) 37, 38, 77.
Genetic map 59.
Genetic polymorphism 31, 38.
Genistein 13, 27, 96, 97, 104, 162.
GGT, see gamma-glutamyl-transferase
Glucosinolates 27, 29.
Glutathion-peroxydase 28, 64, 88, 97.
Gluten intolerance 141.
Glyceride fraction 58.
Gums 97-99.

H

HDL, see high density lipoprotein
Health benefit 3, 39, 53, 70, 77, 78, 93, 94, 100, 103, 113, 141, 143-145, 151.
Hemicellulose 97-99.
Herbs 9, 10, 11, 39, 116, 117, 121, 149.
High density lipoproteins 56, 162, 163.
Hydrocarbons 58, 161.

I

Insulin-resistance syndrome 9, 10, 18, 31, 34.
Intima 79.
Isoflavones 19, 96, 97, 104, 105, 162.
Isothiocyanates 27, 29, 95.

L

Lag time 62, 82, 86.
LDL, see low density lipoproteins
LDL, oxidability of 142.
Leguminous plants 95, 97, 100, 118, 122, 134, 141.
Lignans 17, 19, 20, 97, 163, 164.
Lignin 96-99, 109.
Linoleic acid 35, 55-57.
Lipids
– saturated 54, 110.
Low density lipoproteins 54, 55, 94, 142, 163.
LTB4 70, 87.
Lysine 97, 100.

Index

M

Macrophages 56, 64, 89, 161.
Macular degeneration 29.
Maturity 58, 59, 115, 142.
Meat consumption 9, 29-32, 55, 70.
Mediterranean pyramid 140, 152.
Metal chelators 59.
Methionine 13, 95, 100, 134, 163.
Milk 9, 19, 33, 34, 55, 75, 114, 118, 119, 132, 134, 136, 143, 149.
Mineral elements 96, 97, 131, 134.
MONICA 37, 38, 77.
Monocytes 64, 79, 89.

N

New agricultural practices 139, 140.
Nutrients 3-5, 7, 10, 12, 17, 20, 22, 28-31, 70, 94, 98, 113, 131, 133, 134, 136, 139, 141, 145.
Nutritional density 94.
Nutrition policies 149, 154-158.
Nutritional qualities 136.
Nutritional value 93, 131, 134, 135, 141, 142, 157.

O

Oleic acid 35, 53, 55-57, 65, 142, 143.
Oleuropein 35, 59-61, 164.
Olive 35, 36, 53, 58-62, 64, 65, 82, 94, 104, 105, 115, 119, 123, 142, 151.
Olive oil 9, 11, 35, 36, 53-62, 65, 82, 94, 104, 105, 120, 139, 140, 142, 143, 149, 151, 153, 154, 156, 163, 164.
Osteoporosis 34, 35, 39, 65.
Oxidation resistance 75, 80, 82, 87.
Oxidised LDL 13, 161.
Oxygen reactive species 80.

P

Pectins 97-99.
Peroxidation 32, 94.
Phenolic acids 59, 61, 64, 82, 83, 85, 86, 88, 95, 96, 104, 105.
Phenolic compounds
– chemical structures of the main classes 106.
Phyto-oestrogens 19, 34, 94, 97, 98, 104, 164.
Phytosterols 58.
Polyphenols 13, 27, 53, 57-62, 64, 65, 80, 82-89, 94, 96, 97, 103-105, 136, 142, 145, 149.
Potassium 14, 96.
Preservation conditions 72, 132.
Preservation techniques 72, 122.

R

Recommendations 39, 70, 110, 113, 114, 139, 143, 150, 151, 153, 156-158.
Reducing agents 95.

S

Selection 24, 60, 131, 142.
Selenium 28, 64, 97.
Sodium 96.
Squalene 58.
Starches 118, 123, 139, 140.
Sterols 58.
Sulphur compounds 27, 95.
Sunshine 35, 140.

T

Tannins 87, 96, 100, 104, 105.
Technological treatments 131, 134, 135, 146.
Terpenes 27, 29, 95.
Tocopherols 12, 26, 58, 72, 81, 94, 95, 134, 161.
Traditional Mediterranean diet 76, 109, 113, 150, 151.
Transmethylation 95.
Triglycerides 32, 55, 58, 71, 133, 163, 164.
Triterpenic alcohols 58.

V

Varieties 58-60, 123, 141-143, 151.
Vegetables 7-11, 13-17, 19, 20, 22, 28-30, 35, 36, 39, 58, 65, 74, 93, 94-97, 100, 104,

Index

105, 109, 113-120, 123, 136, 139-142, 145, 146, 149, 151, 154, 162.
Vegetable water 59.
Vitamins 6, 10, 13, 22, 94, 95, 124, 131, 133, 134, 136, 140, 141, 143, 149.
Vitamin B12 13, 94, 95, 136.
Vitamin C 6, 7, 12-15, 20-23, 25-28, 94, 97, 101, 134, 136.
Vitamin E 11-13, 20, 22, 23, 25-29, 35, 36, 58, 62, 64, 72, 81, 82, 87-89, 94, 95, 134, 136, 161.

W

Water content 94, 146.
Wall of a vessel 79.
Water rich products 94.
Wine 7, 9, 37, 38, 58, 77, 78, 82, 84-89, 94, 96, 104, 105, 119, 123, 133, 139, 145, 149, 151-153, 156.

Y

Yoghurts 9, 33, 139, 143, 151.

Achevé d'imprimer par Corlet, Imprimeur, S.A.
14110 Condé-sur-Noireau (France)
N° d'Imprimeur : 54248 - Dépôt légal : novembre 2001

Imprimé en U.E.